Alchemy for Life

Formulas for success

I0130065

MARK BRADFORD

Copyright © 2019 Mark Bradford

Printed in the United States of America
First Printing, 2019

Alchemy

ISBN-13: 978-1-7336622-2-2

Library of Congress Control Number: 2019904364

alchemyfor.life

v1.4

DEDICATION

To everyone who doesn't beat themselves up when they fail.

To all the Alchemists - past, present and future - I dedicate this book to you.

CONTENTS

One

Two: Alchemy & Alchemy For Life

Three: Coaching

Four: Formulas and Goals

Time can go slow for the things you do like.
Productivity is efficiency, and efficiency is proper flow
Efficiency is happiness

Awareness is the first step
The workplace is different

Ups and downs and goals

Let's be real
Rocks and Feathers
Your inertia
Things in motion in your life
Things at rest in your life
Awareness
Your Homework

Cutting the grass and sump pump hoses
Resting and tension?
Tension
Resting

Order or Chaos?
Order
Chaos
You're Both, but when?

Job
Career
Calling
What do you have?
Goals
Alternate routes
It's nonlinear

If you're the canary

Charging a battery
Filling a bucket
Accomplishments and goals
Be mindful

The raising and the dashing
Two things make a huge difference
Dread
Here's what to do about dread

Four: Your hurdles

Worksheets

ACKNOWLEDGMENTS

I'd like to express my appreciation for the people in my life that that have helped me. But there's more to it than that generic statement, because there are people in my life that help me not because I ask, or because they provide a service that I am interested in engaging or purchasing.

No, the people I am thanking are those people who have helped me by making a simple suggestion, or a comment, or given feedback. Those people took time to be simply sincere to me and offer their input or way of doing things. You would be amazed at how a random comment can make a huge difference in the energy you have available to get through something.

A lot of writing is in a vacuous secret world.

So thank you. It meant a lot, even though I didn't let you know it at the time. You probably wouldn't have believed how much it meant to me anyway and shrugged it off.

Because in your eyes, you were just being you.

USING THIS BOOK

I want to help you through this book, and I want you to get the most of out it. A lot of effort and history went into creating it. This book has been very patient so I want to make sure I do a good job of presenting it to you.

You see, my first book was called *The Status Game* and it was about the ups and downs, the annoyances, the hilarious fantasy world of online dating. When it was done I jumped on writing this book. After all I was right in the middle of coaching, and had recently created the Alchemy for Life™ system - the system and the online system that made it all pretty.

But then something happened.

I heard a knocking at my brain. It was more information on *The Status Game*. No, it wasn't an extra chapter or something I had forgotten to include. Instead, it was the realization that with *The Status Game* I had laid the groundwork for something much bigger. If status was a thing, then all these other things were true. Everything about it - how we relate to others, how we see the world - all came together.

But there was a problem. The reason I was able to publish *The*

Status Game was the fact that I put myself through my own coaching. Yes, it is as crazy as it sounds. I did that partially to test the system (I'd done that with others too, but wanted to see it as a "client" first hand). One of the challenges I brought to my "coach" was that I did an awful lot of writing but like so many people I didn't have a book to show for those efforts.

After looking at my balance sheet[1], he told me the following:

Pick one book and stick with it. Write it till it's done. No writing anything else (no other book) until it's done.

That was really hard. What a jerk he/I was.

So that's what I did, and it worked[2].

But that's what also created the problem. So when I started to write this book and another book came knocking I just wrote down the little snippets for later (that's also what the coach suggested[3]). But the snippets turned into sentences and the sentences turned into paragraphs and the paragraphs turned into chapters. I was done. I had to stop working on this book in favor of the other book - it just *demanded* to be written.

That book became *The Status Game II* - a greatly expanded and deep dive into status, the three forms of it, the way we choose friends, the way we choose romantic partners, even where our self-esteem comes from and goes horribly wrong.

Writing and publishing is just the beginning. Book promotion takes on a whole life of its own. During this promotion I started writing a book on something very personal - my view of spirituality, religion and lack thereof. Don't worry - it's written

---

[1] The Balance Sheet is the online, colorful form that helps you lay out where all your time, energy and resources are going.

[2] You could say I definitely practice what I preach.

[3] This is sounding really cray, isn't it?

with the complete understanding that it all may be silly. The first sentence sums it all up so nicely: *Believe it or not, it doesn't matter.* The double entendre is just delicious.

Now that I have published three books I can finally come back to the book that's waited so patiently for me to continue.

Why do you think that happened? From a writing perspective I've found that I don't write things because I want to; I write them because I *have* to. They dictate to me who is next.

I think the other bonus of this book having patience is that it also gave me an opportunity to gather much more wisdom on the topic. After all in the mean time I've produced a Sunday podcast every week and interviewed amazing people from (literally) all over the globe.

So here it is. Thank you for waiting as well.

Truly Self-Help

I wrote this book truly as a "self-help" even though I'm supposed to call it "personal productivity." Call it what you want; it's a self-help book. In being that, it is something that should allow *you* to help *you*.

The smartest way to do that is to break this into four parts. First I am going to tell you what my story is, how I got to the point, the journey I took (or in some cases was forced to take) to get here. How did I get to book four? I do this because you may find we have something in common and even if we don't you'll know that I too struggled. We all do.

Then you will need to know what all this "alchemy" stuff is. It's important that you understand the metaphor and the system. I didn't just create a metaphor but an entire system built around people like you reaching goals. But first I had to understand what life is made of.

In being that, it is something that should allow *you* to help *you*.

Once you understand that, we can discuss coaching. Coaching used to creep me out - not sports coaching, or business coaching - but the coaching of the "life" variety. It doesn't anymore. Not because I do it, but because I understand what *true* coaching is. I've also found out that what I'm doing is a bit different that what other people do - thus the label of "anti-coach." There's a rant in there - useful, emotional and candid.

When you understand and embrace this we can then move forward to you accomplishing goals - the good stuff. Those parts are as follows:

SECTION ONE: My Story - how I got here

One of my first talks was at the headquarters of Manpower, to a room full of C-level professionals that were in transition. Meaning, they were between careers or considering moving from one job to another. It is very important to get feedback, and this talk included feedback forms. As it was one of my first talks I was expecting that the feedback would be in line with that - there would be lots of room for improvement and I'd be informed of that fact clearly. This did not happen; they were very happy with the talk, the subject matter, the delivery, everything. The thing that surprised me more was that more than one person made the comment that I had left something out. I was so focused on providing a framework and imparting wisdom (and not making it a commercial) that I hadn't - according to them - really provided much about my back story.

The reason for this was that I thought the absolutely intense, absurd and almost unbelievable story had no place in the talk.

After all these were very painful, almost embarrassing life trials I had been though. I could have talked about them for hours. As I called the totality of the information, this was a "three martini and large popcorn" kind of discussion.

Yet this wouldn't be the first time people requested more information.

That was a long time ago, and I would go on to write *The Status Game II*[4] in which I spent an entire chapter on vulnerability, because eventually I got it.

So allow me to tell you my story. Perhaps we have some things in common. Perhaps you'll agree with the CEOs in transition, and other audience members - that it is good to hear where someone is coming from.

SECTON TWO: Alchemy & Alchemy for Life

You have probably had your fair share of metaphors; in fact everyone thinks they are The Metaphor Master (I never see them at the meetings though).

So you ask, what is all this "alchemy" stuff and what is this Alchemy for Life™ thing? Is it magic? Is it some sort of system? I will give you an explanation of what Alchemy for Life™ is. Some people may be familiar with "alchemy" and some not. But "Alchemy for Life" is something I created that needs explaining. I'll explain what alchemy is, what it *was* and how I've incorporated it into my view on life (and reaching tangible goals).

SECTION THREE: Coaching

I'll tell you what coaching is and (more importantly) isn't. Everyone's a Life Coach these days it seems. You may be

---

[4] *The Status Game II: Dashboards and Gages.*

surprised at how that term creeps me out. This book is in your hands in place of working with me as a coach. Perhaps we will work together; perhaps we already have. Regardless you'll want to understand what coaching (of the proper life coaching variety) truly is. You may be at the point in which you think this is all nonsense and are about to give up on reaching goals with the help of a coach. That's OK. Really.

SECTION FOUR: Moving forward and reaching your goals.

What good is all this if you don't come away with some tangible, doable stuff? Once we have all this overhead out of the way we can then move on to the tangibles. But if you don't even know what the brake pedal does on a car teaching you how to get to your grandma's house would be useless. Maybe it'd even be dangerous, but at least very frustrating.

I'll help you to see your life as a system (the way I see everything) and help you to make room for goals, instead of just trying to shoe-horn them in. The last half of the book is filled with real world examples on what to do, what not to do, how to do it and what I have encountered. Please don't skip to that section, as you really want to understand the whole Alchemy for Life™ approach and not fall prey to any of the pitfalls that I've already figured out.

In addition, if you start to get a really good handle on things you may find yourself with more time, energy and resources than you had before. This surplus of the three elements of life may put you in an enviable position - you now have to decide what to do with this extra time, energy and resources.

Sounds like a problem most people would embrace.

Systems, not goals

I'm never going to mention goals without affirming solidly that they have to be part of a system. Your goals should always be part of a system so you can actually accomplish them. In the fourth section of the book I'm going to talk about what to do - moving forward - about these goals.

This surplus of the three elements of life may put you in an enviable position - you now have the decide what to do with this extra time, energy and resources.

We will talk about what to expect, what you'll encounter and I'll offer some things for consideration. We will tackle the ups and downs of life, whether that thing you do is a job, career or calling (hint: if all the work you didn't do while on vacation is waiting for you it's more than a job). We will talk about the difference between momentum and inertia, why the way battery chargers (and baristas) work teaches us how finishing a goal is so hard some times.

We will talk about the importance of something most people never consider when pursuing a goal - your job. I'm not talking about a new career *as* a goal, I'm talking about *any* goal.

We will talk about our perception of time and how we can can actually make the enjoyable moments go slower.

Dread and doubt - two of your biggest invisible enemies - will be defeated in one day.

And then comes the new years resolutions - in some cases that has been your only experience ever with setting a life-changing goal.

Spoiler alert - I'm going to tell you not to make them.

Finally there are worksheets at the end of this book. Please use them when the chapters are fresh in your mind. Ideally once you make it through the book you will then be primed for the worksheets. Don't worry, they are very simple but will get you to think about and record things you may never even have considered.

I would not suggest you read a chapter, then jump to the worksheet - I would have included them in their respective chapters if I thought that was a good idea. No, instead, reading through the entire book allows you to understand everything as a whole.

We will go through this together. Ready?

Mark Bradford

Alchemy for Life

MY STORY

It's probably been over ten years since I got divorced. "Got divorced" is such a bland, misleading statement. For so many people this is not only a massively life-changing event, but a very messy emotional thing. The system of marriage is not created with any regard to an end.

After being married for a number of years things changed[5]. This change caused me to be a full-time dad at the same time I was running my little technology business. Up till then my wife was a stay at home mom. Now I was a stay at home dad, that *also* worked full time with full placement of the kids. That was a challenge.

When this happened I didn't take things lightly, and believed I had signed up for good and bad times. So I dug in and did everything I could to save things, for myself and the family unit.

The One thing I can't explain

The lyrics of a song seemed to describe exactly what was

---

[5] I just saved you about 30 pages of reading.

11

happening - before I was aware of what was happening.

Music is a very powerful thing. It's literally a religious or spiritual experience for many people, whether it is a pop song that pulls on their heart strings or a song they associated intensely with a relationship. When the relationship ends the music is still there to remind them of the feelings they once had. It invokes those intense feelings of love, completeness, happiness - even though the reality that created those feelings is no more.

Announcing that a song seemed to be describing your relationship is a given - in fact many songs are designed to do that with fairly generic broad brush strokes of sorrow, of missing someone, etc.

So what I am about to tell you is not a story of associating a feeling with a song, or waxing philosophical because of hearing "our song." This is a song with no connection, no emotional anchor, no hooks. This is an occurrence that I could not explain, and was the start of the worst experience of my life.

When I started my business I stopped using an alarm clock. I, like many people, noticed that I would just wake up right around the time the alarm was set for anyway. So I started experimenting. Yes, I would just wake up at the time I was supposed to and then just get up. I researched this and found a paper explaining why college kids who fell asleep on a bus never missed their stops. They were clearly asleep yet when they reached their stop they would wake up and groggily leave the bus. The explanation was that a part of their brain was never really asleep. You see, they were having "microbursts" of awareness. Their eyes would open a little, their ears would perk up. They learned to recognize the feeling of the bus coming to a stop, the driver saying the stop's street name. In some cases it was the view out the window.

So a part of them was monitoring the progress of the bus and the real world while they slept.

That's what I was doing. I was ahead of the game though. You see, without an internal chronometer, how do you just "wake up" at a certain time?   I wasn't just waking up *around* the time I was supposed to; I was waking up at exactly the minute I was supposed to.   And with some experimenting I could change the time - and wake up at that moment instead.

As a lazy engineer type, I bought a clock that projected the time on the ceiling.   It was completely unnoticeable unless the room was dark - then the large bright red numbers were there, hovering directly above me.

I was able to wake up at whatever time I wanted to because - like the college kids - I was monitoring the external environment and as long as I could see what time it was I could wake up whenever I told myself to.

But then I took it a step further.   What about music?   When I was young I would sometimes fall asleep hearing music.   It seemed I could direct it at times as I drifted off.   So because of that, I wondered what would happen if I also told my internal alarm to "wake me up with music."   So, I picked a song and sure enough the next morning I woke up to the song I requested. Mind you, this was just a few seconds and it immediately subsided once my eyes were opened, but it worked.   I did it a couple times and figured I shouldn't mess around with my brain too much.

The mind is an amazing thing.

What does all this have to do with the most painful time of my life?   It's my attempt to give a scientific explanation to the unexplainable thing that happened.

As I said something serious was going on in my marriage - countless talks, adjustments, etc., revealed dead ends. I signed us up for counseling, assured the kids, took daily walks with them to hear what they had to say.   But something was wrong.

So one day, after weeks of wondering, I went to bed and prayed. I prayed for a long long time before I fell asleep. I said that I would just handle whatever it was, but I just wanted an *answer*. Call it meditating; call it communing. You can read my thoughts on the subject as I wrote a book on it[6].

Regardless, my desperation produced a result.

The next morning a song blasted in my ears - not the subtle internal sounds I was familiar with from the other experiments, this was different. This was loud, clear music that didn't stop even when my eyes were open. I stared at the ceiling and just listened. It was a song I hadn't heard in a long time.

It was "Hold On," by YES.

> *Justice to the left of you*
> *Justice to the right.*

I kept listening. And when the chorus hit me the song ended.

> *Hold on - Hold on*
> *Wait maybe the answer's looking for you.*

I asked for an answer, and was presented with a song whose chorus told me that the answer was looking for me.

That day my wife's friend's husband called and said he wanted to drop my daughter off - she had slept over the night before. The way he said it made me wonder, like he needed me to be home alone.

He did. I was. We talked.

"She's cheating on you, man."

---

[6] *OneSelf: Have faith. In yourself.*

The answer was looking for me, had found me, and had devastated me.

"Forever" was apparently 13 years.

What followed was a long proceeding involving a lot of learning, a lot of pain, a lot of redefining, and a lot of juggling.

Then the surgery happened. Due to a bulging disk[7] I was losing strength in my arm. The doctors involved acted fast and I was scheduled for surgery - on Thanksgiving.

My wife was particularly annoyed at the extra time she had to put in with the kids and getting me to the hospital. Going into surgery, I said "I love you" to her. "I love you too" she replied. I was terrified, but now I had hope.

My daughter desperately wanted to stay over in the hospital - she thought she was going to lose her dad. My wife would not allow it, I later learned.

I was only in the hospital for a day or so, and was sent home missing two disks, but with the addition of one plate, six titanium screws and a neck brace I was to wear for 30 days - including in the shower.

Once home and talking to my wife I repeated the "I love you." She just stared at me. When I tilted my head and asked what was going on she said, "I told you this wouldn't change anything." She had. She told me that this surgery made no difference on how she felt about me. The "I love you" in the hospital had been not for me, but for everyone else in the room.

Each morning I woke up to reality. The neck brace made sleeping difficult; the metal in my neck terrified me and made me feel less of a human. My marriage was over, and the daily screaming that

[7] The cause of this was confusing.

was happening between my wife and my kids was getting worse.

Each morning I faced the ceiling and cried.

But life had to go on. I had to continue and be a good dad. My kids needed me and were going through a very difficult time too. It seemed that one parent was no longer interested in being a parent. The other was in a neck brace. And I still had a business to run, by myself.

I was prescribed a month of heavy pain killers. I took them, dozed off, was sad. The Monday after the surgery I returned to the doctor for the follow-up. I told him I stopped taking the meds - I didn't like how they made me feel. Truth be told I preferred the painful reality to the semi-dream like state the meds were putting me in.

He was surprised. "Then you can drive," he said. It wasn't the neck brace preventing me from driving; it was the meds. And since I had voluntarily ended them after 48 hours, I was good to go.

So, with a clear head I returned to work the next day - in a snow storm. I couldn't turn my head to check my blind spot, so I just put my turn signal on and waited, and hoped. I eventually figured out other ways to approach this[8].

As I eventually came to understand what was happening to me and my kids I decided to take them to a psychologist. Even though I was putting tremendous effort into making sure they had a voice, were as OK as they could be (in the circumstances) I still knew that a third party's view on things would be valuable and necessary - especially with the unusual happenings.

This psychologist was a wonderful woman that interviewed the kids, and me. This was not a court-mandated visit; this was

---

[8] This was before cars that checked your blind spot for you and alerted you to other cars - boy that would have been helpful.

something I voluntarily wanted for the kids. I thought at the time that I would rather them find I was doing something wrong than not. You want what's best for your kids and that desire is not limited by your own selfishness - in theory.

But then she asked me a question:

"But what are you doing for you?'

Things went surprisingly well and after a few visits the psychologist eventually turned her focus on me. She told me I was doing a wonderful job of making sure the kids were good, safe and heard. She said I was surprisingly objective and that it translated into a very healthy environment for the kids. Unfortunately my methodology of proceeding with as little conflict as possible as my marriage dissolved was not going to work. She told me it was a toxic environment and I could not just stand by - I needed to act. So I acted, and went against everything I had planted, and established for ten plus years. Forever was a lot shorter than previously discussed; being a husband and being a parent were at odds.

Priorities had shifted, beliefs were challenged, just standing by and being kind was just not going to work.

When the dust had all settled the psychologist asked me a question:

"But what are you doing for you?"

It was this question that would set me on the path to found Alchemy for Life, start a podcast, and seek out the meaning of balance. And perhaps life?

My response to her was a blank stare, as if someone had unplugged my brain:

File Not Found[9].

The truth is, I wasn't doing *anything* for me. I was focused on these new tremendous, unexpected, unplanned life-changes. The kids were everything, and all of my focus was on them. In *The Status Game II* I discuss the revelation that my "gage" for parenting was set higher than my "gage" for husband. And my gage for being a husband was set pretty high - I liked being a husband. Heavy stuff, but even that had limits. Hit me like a ton of bricks. I remember the feeling I had when I knew I was getting a divorce - it was the saddest feeling I had ever felt in my life by an order or two of magnitude. And then literally a minute or so later that monumentally sad and hopeless feeling was replaced by an even stronger feeling of sadness and failure.

My own kids were going to have divorced parents.

I understand that the divorce rate is fairly close to 50%, and that this fact has become sort of the "norm" but it wasn't to me, however. So all of my energy was in making sure the kids would be OK.

When we fly and are subjected to the mandatory safety demonstration that everyone ignores. When they get to the part about there being a breach and an oxygen issue they tell you that you have to put your mask on first before you put your kids' masks on. That's counter-intuitive. You want to save them. You want to save the kid on the plane and allow them to breathe. But that's backwards.

My own kids were going to have divorced parents.

---

[9] That's what it felt like.

What you need to do is save *yourself* first, then you can save *them*.

The lesson is that if you don't survive you can't take care of your kids. And as the psychologist made clear, if there was nothing left of me I wasn't going to be a very effective dad.

So I put my mask on first and started to figure out what I wanted, in addition to being a dad. Not only did it not take away from my care of my kids, but they saw that I was taking care of myself too and they were quite enthusiastic about it. I learned a lot about their perspective on it.

Balance. The beginnings of understanding was happening.

Then I went out on dates, and so forth. Going out on dates - many many dates - exposed me to the crazy and upside-down world of online dating. That exposure of using the big five dating sites made me analyze how it all worked. So after about a year or so of this I sat down and in a labor of love (quite literally) I created my own dating site from scratch. Since I learned that we make decisions in about seven seconds it seemed that a connection happened in the time span of a glance. Thus I called the new site "Only a Glance."

It seemed to make sense.

I would then go on to write two books about everything I learned dating and how it was all related to something I call *status*[10].

I had to sort out this new life of having my kids full time, running my small business, putting myself out there and dating, and figuring out who I was.

I found that when you are a couple you know who you were together, but when you part you then have to find out who you *are*. We all make concessions and adjustments in a relationship. That is

[10] *The Status Game*, and *The Status Game II*.

not to say that we change and are disingenuous. It means that each relationship imparts changes and wisdom upon us, and we must reflect upon these changes. And wisdom. So when we are between partners we learn a bit more about ourselves. Sometimes we find new interests, new hobbies. My writing did not really kick into high gear until after I was divorced.

A lot of self-reflection happened, as you can imagine. My greatest talent at the time was making it all my fault, my responsibility. I found that if it's your fault then you can control it, change it and make it better. How great is that? Make it all your fault and you can make it all better.

Grow up, Mark.

Unfortunately we have a lot less control than we think. The same was true for me. I couldn't change the course of events - all I could do was make the best of them.

This self-reflection made me think hard about what I was doing with my life. I was writing fiction, building a dating site, I had created a role-playing game, was coding applications online, even giving talks to kids about writing, and running a tiny tech company helping local businesses with their technology needs.

Grow up, Mark.

That's what I said to myself, in a moment of maximum irritation. I'd been running my business for over ten years while doing all these other things.

Grow up and maybe get a real job. Stop all the entrepreneurial nonsense. No one in my family, or friends at the time were like that. My bestie had worked at a law firm immersed in corporate America doing the same job for his entire life. I could always hear him glaze over when I told him about what I was doing - like I was on another planet.

I could just stop all this stuff and get a real job, a job with vacation and sick time and a retirement fund and actual insurance that didn't cost a fortune and deliver nothing.

But then something very interesting happened. While having talks with a lot of people I went down the path of figuring out what my core talents were. Core talents are the things or thing that makes you you - the thing that you do pretty well. Your purpose, if you will.

Well, my "purpose" wasn't to make role-playing games, it wasn't to write fiction or non-fiction, it wasn't to give talks, or code web applications, or find technological solutions for clients and explain them in English. It wasn't to build dating sites or make snarky card games to challenge the whole concept of finding a mate. And it wasn't to coach people to find goals.

It was all of those things.

My core talent is to see things from a perspective that most people do not see, and to build, augment, fix or create a system to address that.

In other words, look at something, and come up with a system to make it better. And explain it nicely.

Thats my core talent. And that's what had been driving me all this time. RPGs were clumsy so I created one in which special dice did all the work. Online dating was all wrong, so I built a dating site to address that, and wrote a book about it.

My core talent is to see things from a perspective that most people do not see, and to build, augment, fix or create a system to address that.

Relationships seemed to follow a set of invisible rules, so I wrote two books about that. And created a card game.

Coaching was so linear, didn't look at the big picture[11], and lacked a specialized visual tool, so I created a system and built a tool online.

And businesses had needs so I came up with and built unique and friendly ways to address them.

Two core skills, guiding me and aiding me.

Now you know how I got here. Perhaps your story is similar?

Let's figure out these goals and this balance together. And in the process maybe we can figure out your core skills too.

---

[11] As in, it was not "holistic."

Mark Bradford

THE THREE ELEMENTS OF LIFE

I thought long and hard about what life was really made of. Surely it was made of millions of different things - each unique and undefinable. To my minor surprise I found I was able to narrow it down (this ability to define things in simple terms - distilling in a way that made sense and was easy to demonstrate - was something I now understand as my core talent, as I mentioned previously. At the time I was just becoming aware of this ability.)

Life is not a box of chocolates, nor is it a cereal that's not too bad unless you let it get soggy in the milk for too long. No, it's just three things: Time, Energy and Resources. That's it. Everything you do is made of at least one of those things. And more often than not you are giving away two or more of them.

For example, when you go to your job you give up time and energy, but you get back resources (in the form of your paycheck). You also get some deferred time and energy in the form of vacation and sick time. Did you ever think of it that way? Probably not.

No, it's just three things: Time, Energy and Resources. That's it.

Energy can take many forms. It's not just physical energy, but there is mental stamina and emotional gas to consider. Too much? Don't worry, I'll break it all down for you. That's my job[12].

Let's revisit energy a little later, and instead address it in the order I like to say it, "Time, Energy and Resources."

Time

We all get that, right? There's only so much time in the day, we all get the same amount and it passes whether we do anything or not. Pretty basic.

Or, one would assume. The truth is that time is largely perception. Sure, it takes a fixed amount of time to properly make meringue cookies, or for a plant to grow, or to complete a master's degree. However, the *passage* of time is fluid, and an experience vs. a set function of realty. Wow, what the heck does that mean, right?

It means that the same hour of time can have a distinctly different meaning, feeling and speed of passage for one person over another. A task completed by you can take agonizingly long, but for someone else it can zip by. Doesn't matter how we "feel" about an hour because it's the same damn hour you say? Oh but it does, as we experience life through our perception and feelings. This ever-growing and changing filter is not only how we experience time, but how we *remember* it.

The truth is that time is largely perception.

Time is a fluid thing. Much more on this later.

---

[12] That core skill.

Energy

There are actually three kinds of energy. Stay with me. Why is that important? Because each kind of energy allows you to do something special. And, you may have a lot of one, but not much of the other two. And finally, some activities use one kind of energy but not the other two, while other activities may use all three.

Physical Energy

It takes energy to exercise, to do a yoga class, to run a marathon, to chase toddlers around and to be a landscaper. We all get that. If you are tired from doing any of that it's quite visible in the form of sweating, looking like you need some water and just having that "I just ran a marathon" look in your eyes.

Mental stamina

But there's more to energy than that. If you have a non-physical office job like so many of us unfortunately have, then you aren't using up much *physical* energy. However, if you are tasked with managing large projects, juggling many clients and treating them like they are the *only* clients, or running your own business - regardless how small - then you expend a lot of mental energy. Your brain can be quite tired at the end of the day.

If you don't have that kind of job you've probably still been exposed to that by going to a work party[13], or sitting down with an attorney or a tax professional. You expend a lot of mental energy.

What happens then?

---

[13] "work" parties are much more taxing than regular parties. You have to be "on" all the time.

27

Emotional Gas

Some us go through life in a bubble - we have very few ups and downs and the family for the most part behaves itself. However there are those of us that have had some pretty emotionally trying times. Going through a divorce - messy or not - having to deal with a life-changing event, an illness that's just not going away, or caring for a loved one with complicated needs are all things that can be quite taxing emotionally.

If you are running a marathon you are for the most part just using physical energy right? If you go to work out, again, just physical energy right?

Nope.

If it's just physical energy, then think about the last time you wanted to work out and didn't: was it because you didn't think your legs could run on that tread mill?

Uh oh. Truth time. No, I doubt seriously that anyone who avoids working out and then feels guilty about it ever avoided it because they assessed themselves physically and said "I don't think my muscles can lift that 30 times, or run on the elliptical for 20 minutes."

Instead it was something else - you didn't *feel* like it. Feel? Yep, that's emotional gas. Some people may tell you that's a "mindset" and lots of other motivational yet fairly useless things. Call it whatever you want; but it's the emotional energy that managed whether you went or not.

Think about that. If it was only a physical limitation you would be extremely fit. If you went and worked out every time you wanted to (assuming you had the time and resources) then you would be in exceptional physical shape. The people who do succeed in doing that are those that master the emotional side of it.

Think about that. If it was only a physical limitation you would be extremely fit.

You kind of knew that, you just never heard it spelled out like that.

Again, "I don't feel like working out" does not equal "My body is incapable of performing the physical activity I have planned." Sure you can't just walk into a gym and lift, and run and perform things that you just decide to do. Obviously there are indeed physical limitations. But if you have the membership, or the bike, and the time to do it and you say "I'm going to go spend an hour being physical" what is stopping you? Your emotion is, of course.

Resources

Resources seems like a pretty simple thing - it's just stuff you have to spend. Your bank account and the stuff you possess are your resources. That's all right? Sort of. As I said when you give up your time and energy to your job, career or calling you presumably get resources back in the form of cold hard cash. This cash is then used to pay for other resources you purchase from the government and private businesses - natural gas, electricity, gasoline, clothing, etc.

You also accumulate resources that you can use for other things, or even trade with others. If you own a car you have a car you can lend to a friend. If you have a house you can rent out (or lend out) a room to someone. Even two women trading outfits because they are the same size and have the same awesome fashion sense are an example of resources.

Now you understand what life is made of.

ALCHEMY

Allow me to explain what "Alchemy" is.

I've always been fascinated with the concept of "alchemy." It's sort of like chemistry, but a bit more mystical and magical. Sir Isaac Newton, who is widely recognized as one of the most influential scientists of all time, laid the foundations for classical mechanics. He worked on hard math and real mechanics of existence.

What a lot of people do not know is that of all of his writings, over a tenth of them are focused on alchemy and the pursuit of the philosophers stone.

When we hear the word "alchemy" we think of people who are almost wizards, concocting things in colorful laboratories, creating flasks of liquids that have properties beyond science. We think of the men in the 17th century who wrote papers on the magical properties of certain elements, and we think of the philosopher's stone.

The Philosophers Stone

According to Wikipedia the philosophers stone was mentioned as far back as 300AD. It represents a mystical undiscovered substance that has all sorts of amazing properties. One of them is to turn base metals to gold. So, somehow exposing lead to it would turn the lead to gold. Seems like a very valuable substance.

In addition it also supposedly had the ability to allow the alchemist to create an elixir of life.

Newton, a man of science, spent an awful lot of his time, energy and resources on researching and discovering this item.

As far as we know he never found it.

What Alchemy is to me

To me "alchemy" is the managing and mixing of things that have seemingly magical properties. The work is part science, part art. By its nature you can never fully understand the works, but you can do your best to do some amazing stuff with it.

Why do I explain alchemy and Sir Isaac Newton's obsession with it? Because like Newton I like lots of neat formulae that make sense. I like things to add up and think the world has a certain order to it[14]. I believe that one can figure out not just the mechanics of relationships as I did in *The Status Game II*, but that you can also figure out the mechanics of life. And like *The Status Game II*, just figuring it out doesn't mean you automatically master it - it means you *begin* to understand.

To me "alchemy" is the managing and mixing of things that have seemingly magical properties.

---

[14] So I call this being "dual-brained" and talk about this in my podcast.

So to me Alchemy has always been a very colorful and amazing concept. I feel that life is made of alchemy - part science and part art. If it was all science you could just write down the stuff you want to accomplish and they would get done. If it was all art then chaos would abound and we'd never develop tools to be better people. It's both.

Alchemy and the flask metaphor

Imagine that life is made of three things - time, energy and resources. Each is a glowing liquid. The time is a pearly white, the energy is blue and the resources is a clear liquid with lots of flecks of gold suspended in it.

Yes? Easy to visualize?

Imagine that each one of us has a big flask - like the one pictured on the front cover. That flask is filled with all three liquids and they swirl around a lot but never mix - like oil and water.

This represents the time, energy and resources in your life.

Imagine that the things that request (and sometimes demand) your attention in life are other flasks - smaller flasks. These smaller flasks represent things like your family, your job, your hobbies, your needs, your desire to exercise, the time you spend dating or building a business. Even caring for a child or pet is a flask.

Every day you take your flask and pour some of the time, energy and resources into these other flasks.

Perhaps some are really huge flasks that need to be contributed to every day; perhaps some are the size of a water truck and you could never fill it up in a day but instead you must contribute some each day (or when you can). This contribution slowly builds over time - like the daily effort it takes to raise a child, or build a career or launch a business, or complete a rather involved piece of art. Or even write a book. They all take some combination of Time, Energy and Resources.

This means that you have a finite amount of time, energy and resources to offer to the various things and people in your life. Of course you do - there's only so much of you to go around. If you look at it this way - like a tangible flask you hold in your hands - you can see how precious these magical liquids are. Because, if you pour out some of your time, you have less time for something else. The same is true for energy and resources.

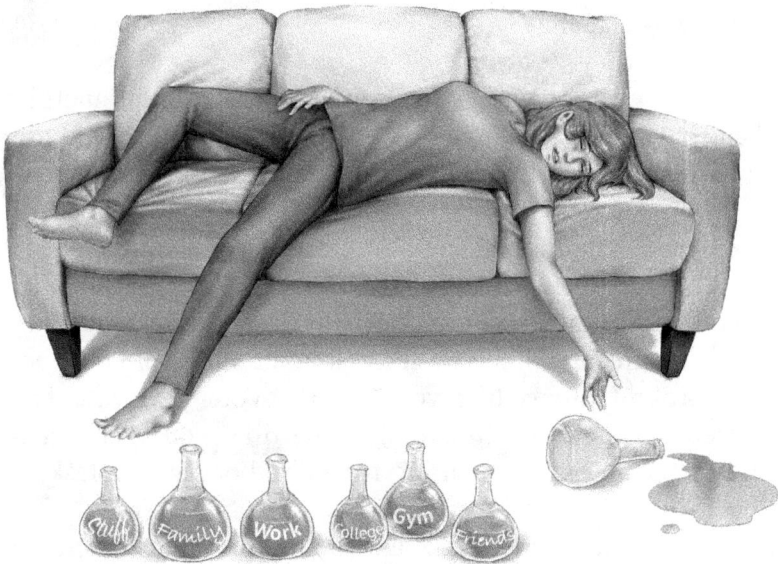

Above: Managing your time, energy and resources can be difficult.

Replenishing your flask

Though you can empty your flask at the end of every day (and sometimes before that!) your flask refills the next day. This refilling of the flask is not always the same; sometimes you don't get the same amount of energy or resources. Sometimes you don't get the same amount of time - because it's still tied up somewhere else.

Kind of like auto-pay, the time is gone before you can even use it.

If you commit to pouring a certain amount of time into something every day - like a job, or caring for a family member - then that time is already gone at the beginning of the next day. Kind of like auto-pay, the time is gone before you can even use it. This is also true for commitments on your energy and resources. Is your paycheck yours, or is a lot or most of it already promised to someone else? Can you do whatever you want on a Tuesday, or did you already promise eight hours to your job, and three hours to your kids? How much energy does it require to care for a toddler? You have that promised and even more.

If only it was so simple that you'd get a flask each morning that was identical to the one yesterday, with 100% of the magical liquids restored.

And each morning you could decide what to do with it - the *whole* thing![15]

But you do not. A lot of your time, energy and resources are already spoken for. You can imagine that those portions are already gone, or that you just pour out the proper amount each day - like a robot, or a servant, or a very responsible adult. You tell me which one best describes you.

---

[15] That's actually what vacation is like for a lot of people. But life isn't vacation.

What if you want to get a dog -or slightly more demanding - a child?

You can see how very important it is to know how much is in the flask, and how much is spoken for.

Because if you don't, then what do you think happens when you want to do something new? What if you want to start a new hobby (or revisit an old one you had to abandon)? What if you want to start dating, or *are* dating but want to see that great person more? What if you want to get a dog - or slightly more demanding - a child.

You would have to do something a surprisingly small amount of people do - you have to check the flask to make sure there is enough left!

That sounds so simple yet so few people do it. They just figure it out. They just make it work. They will find a way.

But seldom they do, because life doesn't really work that way. A good example are the millions of people who buy a gym membership as part of a New Year's resolution because they are "just going to work out regularly" and then before Valentine's Day they stop going. Not because they lack commitment, but because they never made the time for it.

Yes, I recognize that sometimes people take a stand, draw a line in the sand and make an abrupt change when they have a life-changing event. But I am talking about the vast majority of people who want to make a change.

That includes me and *you*.

You have to check the flask first.

But now you understand where "Alchemy" came from, and the flask metaphor.

Now let's apply it.

THE FIVE FACETS OF LIFE

So, now that we know we all have our flasks, and that life is made of Time Energy and Resources, what do we spend it on? Surely there are millions of things to spill our magical liquid into (and receive some in some cases) right? Yes. However, when I asked my core skills about this, they came up with the five facets of life: Spirituality, Health, Rejuvenation/Fun, Learning and Productivity/Obligation. These facets are laid out on something I call The Balance Sheet.

Let's define them so you can understand better.

Spirituality

This is the tangible intangibility, the extra special dimension of life that you can't buy at a store directly (though some may try to convince you otherwise). For some people this is attending their church or temple weekly and participating in the congregation. For others this may be private meditation, others may meditate in groups. Still others may find spirituality in gardening and having zen moments while others find that a bike ride in the country is so unimaginably pretty that they are recharged by the beauty of nature. For many this is yoga. One person may consider that certain music makes them so reflective, so peaceful that it is a spiritual experience - and it doesn't have to be chanting. Someone I know very well feels this way about the music of Jerry Goldsmith.

It's very different for each person, and each one is just as valid[16].

Health

Things that are done for health reasons make the person feel healthy. No surprise there. For some people this is a physical activity such as working out at the gym, dance class, riding a bike, taking a hike, participating in a group sport. Healthy cooking would also go in this column. For others there is a mental component, or it can be solely mental - ever hear of a "healthy attitude?" This is a good opportunity to mention yoga, since for many this can be both spiritual and health-related. It demonstrates that activities can be in more than one facet of life, and many are. You'll usually find that your most meaningful activities are multifaceted.

Rejuvenation/Fun

The good stuff, the juicy stuff, the fun stuff.

As with many of the facets, one person's fun can be another person's work (Productivity/Obligation). You may be rejuvenated by having a drink with a friend, or a girl's night out. Reading may rejuvenate others - a good book may be chicken soup for the... well, you know. Extroverts may really get a charge out of being around people and being in a crowd. Some may be crazy enough to get a kick out of speaking in front of an auditorium of people.

---

[16] See OneSelf: Have faith. In yourself. if you'd like to know my take on it.

Some people are both intro and extrovert I've found. They may enjoy being with people, but then really enjoy the alone time afterwards. Cooking with your partner can be a very romantic activity and very meaningful. So, healthy cooking with a partner would be both fun and healthy. Another crossover. I worked with a client specifically to find her fun, since she was so good at filling the other columns. A lot of movers and shakers - Type A and C level execs - are like this.

Learning

I consider everyone to be life-long learners, even if they don't themselves. We are learning, hopefully, every day. I count things such as reading and researching on the Internet (hopefully dual and triple-sourcing and not just reading your Facebook feed). Reading an article - online or not - counts. Grabbing a book on a subject, taking an Italian Cooking Class, listening to a seminar, even a sermon - all learning. Learning keeps the mind sharp, and open. The more we learn the more we know we don't. Don't *know* that is. Challenging your ideas often can help you better understand yourself, and expose you to things you may never have considered.

Productivity/Obligation

These are the things that we must do (or feel we must do - how it makes you feel is just as important). Obvious obligation items are things like your job, your need to drive your kids to sports (as previously mentioned), perhaps caring for a loved one. Though being a parent is extremely fulfilling and meaningful, there is a certain level of obligation there. Even having a pet, or managing a pool in your back yard is an obligation. There's an obligation component to many things in our lives - even things that may be fun. Then there's the productivity. We are all told to be productive and "productive members of society." You may argue as to the actual productivity of your particular job, but *feeling* productive is a good feeling. We all need that. As previously mentioned, movers and shakers and Type A's usually excel at filling this column. It's usually amazingly long. Then they look at the other columns on the balance sheet and no longer wonder why they are tired, and don't have any energy.

This is part of life and not a bad thing. In fact, if you remove the feeling of productivity from someone, it can have very real effects - very real negative effects[17]. Thus is the case with some retirees. Any job you've ever enjoyed almost certainly had a good component of productivity to it. Cleaning your basement, your closet, gardening, weeding, even working out can feel productive. Helping your scout with his Eagle project, leading the choir at church, feeding the hungry, making dinner - all productive.

Can you think of the things in your life that you spend Time, Energy and Resources on? What did you do today? What is your average Tuesday like?

If you've had a transition then you've probably had to shift, remove or add things to your columns on the sheet.

Can you mentally fill out your Balance Sheet right now?

These facets all describe where you pour your flask. Now that we know where we are pouring it, what then?

Well, that's what balance is all about.

---

[17] Read *The Four Hour Work Week* by Tim Ferris. He touches on how retirement in the traditional sense is not a good thing.

Mark Bradford

ALCHEMY FOR LIFE™

Allow me to explain what "Alchemy for Life™ " is.

Knowing that life was made of Time, Energy and Resources, and understanding that we spend it on five facets of life helped to crystalize what was happening.

If *alchemy* is the mixing and dealing with magical substances to produce amazing results, then doing that same with the liquids that make up life (Time, Energy and Resources) and combining them to accomplish things in the five facets was clearly creating your own alchemical formulas... for your own life.

Thus, seeing your life as a system, knowing that you have finite amount of stuff to spend on it, and understanding how to manage it is clearly Alchemy for Life. So my coaching, my system and this book being based on these principals is known as that. It's not just "making room for stuff in your life" or "watching how much energy you have left" or "you can't play the piano because you don't have time because you do all the caregiving for your kids and your husband needs to do more" or "do you really want to up your handball game or is it that you just want to socialize more."

It's mixing all those things together, respecting that everything requires some combination of the three elements of life, that there's only so much to go around, that your flask gets refilled to a degree and that reaching a goal without a system is not going to work.

It's a way to manage your life, your goals, your energy level, your relationships. It's a way to see where all your time is going, why you don't have any energy, why you should maybe change careers.

It's a clear explanation of why you feel empty lately and how to find the fulfillment of productivity that makes you happy.

It's all that, and more. It's complex, but not complicated.

It's Alchemy for Life™.

Mark Bradford

BALANCE

So what is balance? It sounds sort of boring. It sounds like things are in equilibrium; never changing, always constant. Like a scale. What fun is that?

That's not balance.

The one constant in life is change - things are always changing. We are always changing, adjusting and adapting. As with everything, what is true balance for one person would not be balance for another. Some people may need a lot of fun to offset a small amount of productivity, some may learn on their job and not really need or pursue outside learning. Balance is an individual concept, which is why it lends itself to coaching so well. So how do you know when you have it? Because it makes you feel the following way:

This is balance

You're happy, and content. You feel challenged but not overwhelmed. When life throws you a curve you have the energy to deal with it. You don't spend a lot of time wondering what would happen if you worked out more, or if you're eating really crappy food for the umpteenth day in a row. You don't envy those people who do that thing you want to do. Your balance sheet doesn't have an extra long column and hardly anything in the other columns.

You feel healthy, and productive, and fulfilled. You don't feel guilty about pursuing fun because you're productive. You don't feel like all you do is work out because you're also learning. You feel alive.

That's balance. It's ever-changing because you are, and it's really fun.

The Automation of Balance

You've heard me talk about how as we go through life - especially through our trials and challenges and hardships - we make adjustments. Sometimes those adjustments are extreme or seem out of balance, but at the time they are what we think we need to adjust and get through it. Most of those decisions are minute and subconscious. In fact, that's what most balance is - automated, minute, subconscious decisions.

> That's balance. It's ever-changing because you are, and it's really fun.

Like walking, eating and breathing it's just something we do every day. We don't think about it. We should, because when we leave it on autopilot too long that's when we become imbalanced. Even the aforementioned activities above can become imbalanced if not revisited and refined once in awhile. Take the obvious one - eating. We all know what happens when we just eat - without thinking about it. You're someone who eats sensibly, reasonable portions, fairly often and keeps their blood sugar up, but not too high. Perfect. What could go wrong? Well, now you're working 12 hour days, or on the road a lot so you can no longer pack a healthy lunch. You eat Airport Food, or drink five cups of coffee and destroy your appetite. You go many hours before eating again, then devour something because "all of a sudden" you're starving. Then you eat too much, too fast. You justify because you're working hard. The cycle repeats and you're now feeling unhealthy, have no energy and not exactly thrilled by what you see in the mirror.

Now you get a new job, you're back to being able to pack a lunch, eat reasonably and more often for good blood sugar. But you don't. You find it difficult to pack a lunch. You go out to eat at lunch almost every day and you choose big portions. Why? Because you're eating is still on autopilot. In fact you don't even notice this. I've said before that we go through trauma, changes (divorce, transition, etc.) and we make changes - big changes sometimes. Most of the time they are reactionary, impulsive changes. I don't mean impulsive as in grabbing the Snickers from the check-out line next to the US magazine. I mean impulsive as in a quick reaction to a situation to avoid pain, to adjust to what life's thrown at you. Sometimes you learn it wasn't a good decision, sometimes you don't care because it's better than it was and is a stopgap measure. Sometimes it works, well.

When we make our decisions to adjust and compensate - like new taxes - they don't really come with an expiration date; they just keep going and going. If we don't turn them off they never will stop. You can imagine that some of the things we do to compensate, made with the best of intentions - things that worked really well at the time - can be detrimental to you when the event is over. And that's best case scenario! It can be much worse if you chose a life-changing alteration in your habits or activities to protect you - to adapt, to survive. It can be something that is seriously draining you of Time, Energy or Resources.

Reactive vs Mindful

What do you do then? The first step is to become aware of what you're doing. When my clients fill out the AFL Balance Sheet and work with me they become aware of these adaptations - some do instantly just by seeing the sheet. In fact some soon-to-be clients get that "look" when I describe the Balance Sheet, showing me an awareness they already are developing - and probably why they thought to seek out a balance coach.

If you exercise regularly, you will become aware of your health, your strengths and some of your weaknesses. It's the same for your balance. If you become mindful of how you are balancing your life, you will catch these automatic changes and then grab control.

In my talk on Balance Through Transition I tell people that sometimes when going through a transition they feel they are being pulled along - they are along for the ride. A divorce, a job change, downsizing, an illness - like being placed on a bus and looking out the window. It's a pretty helpless feeling sometimes.

I say grab the wheel.

Run up there and grab the wheel! You may not be able to stop the bus, but you can drive it. At least sit in the chair and fake it. Wave. Play with the radio, adjust the seat. It's much more empowering to grab the wheel and just *own* it. Yep, I'm no longer working. Yep, I have this illness to deal with. But more than anyone else, I'm in control of it. I'm the one making the decisions now on what my next step is in the job search. I'm the one in control on how this illness is handled. I talk about it first. I'm the driver.

At least sit in the chair and fake it. Wave. Play with the radio, adjust the seat.

Yes it makes all the difference in the world, so much so that you will more than once forget you are going through a transition. Why? Because it feels right. An uncomfortable transition is suddenly a life decision that you are doing.

"It's the same damn thing!" you say. "All semantics!" you cry. "No, it's not," I say calmly back to you, and offer you a snack because you're getting crabby.

You're now aware, you're now holding onto the wheel and testing, and annoying the bus that thought it was some sort of automated tour-vehicle. You sit there and hold on to the wheel firmly. As soon as you feel it give a little you start turning. And even when you turn the wheel in the direction it was going to go anyway it was *your* decision.

That's mindfulness, that's being aware and that's being in tune with the automation of balance.

What is "balance coaching?"

Understanding balance now, you wonder what being "coached" to have balance is like, right? Is it beneficial, is it for me?

We should put that question on hold and make sure we are on the same page on half of that - *coaching*.

COACHING

Life Coaching and The Creepometer

Every time I heard that someone was a "Life Coach" my creepometer[18] went up to about nine. I would muse that no one would know that much about "life" and that they couldn't just coach it. You'd have to know so much, like, you know - everything. You'd have to live to be 100+ years old or be an exceptional individual - the likes of which would be extremely rare on this planet. In my talks, this is where I put up a picture of Gandhi, and then Yoda, and everyone laughs. It's true though; this is what would go through my head: some sort of Super Life Master Guy.

But I was wrong. Well, for the most part. I was wrong that a Life Coach was someone with infinite knowledge about life. Granted, there are those that take this lightly, and don't truly get it. But I got it. Once I saw what coaching really was, the value was amazing to me.

---

[18] *Creepometer* is "creep ahmeter," not "creep-o-meter." This measures how creepy or unnerving something makes you feel, not the intensity of a Creep.

What is a coach?

A coach is someone that has your best interests in mind. They are a person you *hire*[19] to allow you to get to a goal of some kind. Blah blah blah. That description just makes you think of a cheerleader to which you pay a lot of money. That's not what a coach is.

Forget every conception you have about what a coach is and remember this one sentence: **A coach is like a spotter at a gym**. You've seen those guys (or gals) - they stand right by the person lifting weights, at a really good angle, and watch. They grab the bar when needed, and they help them complete a rep, and encourage them when they almost quite can't make it. They're not stronger, they're just standing from a different angle.

They have a different perspective.

And, they hold the person accountable to the most important person imaginable - the person lifting the weights.

You.

You are doing the work. *You* are reaching the goals. All of the goals are *your* goals. The coach helps you get there. But don't get caught up on goals.

Forget every conception you have about what a coach is and remember this one sentence: **A coach is like a spotter at a gym**.

Realizing those facts made me see just how valuable a coach was and I suddenly wanted a whole bunch of coaches in my life -

---

[19] This is an important distinction. It is emphasized for a reason.

because it was all good. It was tangible - a tangible service with a measurable deliverable. But I wanted coaches that did it the right way. And the right way had little to do with letters after their names, or tests they'd taken, or group pats on the back by their peers.

Also, I like (and need) tangible stuff. I'm not about the fluffy, foo-foo stuff. Sure it's great to give warm fuzzies to someone, but motivational posters only go so far. I need to have a deliverable, I need to put a handle on it. I'm all about the ... yeah, I'm going to say it again ... *tangible*. I bet you are too.

So I had to think about what I was actually doing, and the best way to do it. How do I make it truly tangible, I asked my core skills. And I had to think about Life, The Universe and Everything[20]. Or at least what life was?

Now that I know what a coach is I have to figure out:

• Life
• How to coach someone in a tangible way

And you know that my core skills answered.

Mark Bradford: The Anti Coach

I've been called this by myself and other human beings. It is a title I wholeheartedly accept - not because I am the opposite of my true concept of a coach, but because I am the opposite of what so commonly passes for a coach.

I do not mean to disparage; I mean to clarify and assert. What I mean by that is I am not calling into question the various flavors and personalities of coaches; they all bring something unique to the table. What I am drawing a distinction on (and therefore accepting the title of "anti-coach") is the definition and

---

[20] I love Douglas Adams.

requirements of what a coach actually is.

Coaching is a business. Businesses have a bottom line. A coaching business is a service-oriented business - meaning that it exchanges time and skill for money. Part of the standard business model for a service-oriented business is to provide samples, consultations and a lucrative long term contract.

That last one doesn't seem to be related to helping you, does it?

Coaching is a business. Businesses have a bottom line.

Let me expand on my observations in this field. Allow me to address the coaches that aren't coaching, directly. The next chapter is not directed at you, but instead *them*. You're along for the ride. If you've encountered anything like this then this will help you to see what's really happening, and keep you from crashing your ship onto the metaphorical rocks.

If you've already sought out coaching and this has been your experience you may have a terrible sinking feeling while also feeling a sort of validation for what you went through.

I do hope that you will be reading this before you experience it, thus preventing you from experiencing it at all. I want your eyes to be open.

What follows is rather outspoken.

If you feel you get what proper coaching is, and we are in agreement on this, then you can spare yourself from the next two chapters/rants. They are my way of being very firm about individuals who help you and those that do not.

Mark Bradford

THE SIRENS OF SELF-HELP

They are all wrong

Are *you* one of *them*? Then you're going to be offended. You're going to say just how wrong I am, you're going to become very defensive and you're going to attempt to cite examples. Then you'll read further and your examples will mostly fall apart. Your further defensive measures will kick in and you will dissect what I am saying. Then you'll peruse my articles, my podcasts, my pages. You'll skim for key words and stuff like that because you're not really the type to read anything thoroughly. You're not about *empirical* data – doubtful you are familiar with the "e" word anyway – and operate mostly on intuition. Everything you do is an emotional reaction to something in your life that was messed up and you're just making this up as you go and trying to project your stuff on everyone else anyway. You're like that, and it has served you well because of your prey.

Unless you are not one of them

Unless you're *not* one of them, and instead you're *the people they attract*. Then we still have time. If you've become tainted, become interested and like the sailors of olde your ship is being drawn to the jagged rocks of stupidity, reactionary narrow-minded logic and fluff due to your despair and frustration then allow me to stand in the way and put a stop to that. No, I'm not going to immediately direct you to my island of logic, systemic approaches, understanding and ultimate tranquility of accomplishment. I first just want to stop your ship from being disintegrated and you from being cast into the ocean of confusion where you sink deeper and deeper into sadness and hopelessness.

The Sirens of Self-Help

What am I talking about? I'm talking about the sirens of self-help – the people who sing their sweet song of I Know Better Than You and If This Happens Do That and also I'm Really Attractive and Have Nice Teeth.

See, a long time ago before science and the scientific method took a solid foothold in our collective intelligence people would rise to notoriety because they noticed a thing. Once they noticed a thing they would then talk this thing up and explain your ills with it. And when that thing made no sense in a particular situation? They'd make up another thing. Yes, make up. You breathed bad air, so we have to make you breathe good air, and let me get the leeches. Feel better now? Sorry about having to remove your leg but hey, that was necessary. Why? Come back in a few days and I'll have an explanation. Also that will be 150 silver pieces, your majesty, and now I'm in Spain. Bye.

The scientific method

The scientific method says essentially come up with a system, test it, test it again and then show it to your peers. Ask "What's wrong with this?" You yourself test it for integrity and for validity. You yourself become a skeptic of your own creations and theories. It's an awfully good method to get some concrete, helpful stuff out there. It's not perfect, and sometimes it makes it hard for "radical'"theories to get much notice but no one's getting leeches in the process.

Their process

Their process – and when I say "their" I mean the aforementioned
Sirens of Self Help – is the opposite, much like the leech providers
of olde. Their method is the opposite of the scientific method.
And much like the providers of olde they focused heavily on the
pains. Have a pain? Do this. See ya. It's a very lucrative
process. It's simple, works for a lot of people and requires very
little other than two things – a little intuition and some confidence.
It doesn't hurt if you are the right gender, age and are attractive.
There's a reason that the sirens are mostly younger, attractive
women. Because it works. I won't go into the details of why, or
why those same principles apply to real-estate agents,
spokespeople, recruiters and salespeople in general. It's a universal
appeal that works on men and women.

I'm in no way detracting from younger attractive women with
charisma, I'm saying that this combination is perfect for a Siren of
Self-Help, because that's all they need: charisma. And of course
there are men sirens. Lots of them.

Identifying them

Which ones are the Sirens? There are some really really great
people out there helping others. But there are indeed a few that are
Sirens. How do you identify them then? Here's how to identify
them and stop your ship from being pulled to the jagged rocks and
the resulting frustration and anger. The following are common
phrases and their translations:

- ***Now is the time for you to do just do it/seek
  adventure.*** Purchase my services! Do it fast while you are
  in a heightened emotional, needful state before you come to
  your senses. This is repeated constantly on their web sites,
  their memes and posts.
- ***Don't let them steal your dreams.*** When your friends and
  family question why you are handing them all that money
  ignore their common sense. Just do it!

- ***Here's what to do when that thing happens.*** They have a common sense thing for you to do, it is incredibly obvious and granular. If you asked yourself the same question you'd say the same thing, but because they said it with a big pretty smile you are going to do it. Never mind that it may not work and you can't really use it again.
- ***Here's how the 'other' people are*** – Typically used by relationship people explaining in detail about a SIDE of the equation. It's always the side on which you are not, which makes it easy to demonize them since you're on the other side. Meaning, here's how "men" are and here's what "women" do.
- ***Blah blah blah leads to happiness*** – They are going to appeal to your desire to be happy. Never mind that only you know what makes you happy, and that the very thing standing in your way might be you, and without figuring out what/why it's never going to change.

OK, so what's my deal

So you ask what my deal is and how I am not a siren? Clearly I am putting effort into deflecting you from them to me right? Well, no not directly. See, I'm not good at marketing. I'm not a fan of the "click funnel" or the "sales funnel." I'm not big on giving out a three page useless PDF that just pats me on the back that is filled with links and thanks for your email because now I'm going to email you constantly until you buy something or shoot yourself or both[21]. This is why my site(s) and my books are filled with information. This is why I have over 50 podcasts, each and every one of them containing more than one tangible takeaway that you can actually use. None of them are overly granular do this tiny thing when this tiny thing happens kind of thing.

---

[21] Literally as of this writing I have just sent up this exact thing - a pop up comes up, you join my mailing list and you get a PDF. In this case it's a five page PDF on what to consider before hiring a coach. Hypocrite or honest? I think the PDF is useful?

Systems are everything

I'm all about systems – I always have been. I didn't realize that until recently but I had always had that focus. I wrote about how our resilience and our ability to deal with tough stuff in our lives *is a system*. I wrote that New Year's resolutions won't work if they are just an empty promise. They work *when there is a system in place* to make them work. When I created the Alchemy for Life™ coaching *system* I not only created a *system*, but literally an *online visual system* that allows people to see the process.

So when I approach how people connect to each other, how relationships – business and personal – work, I see it *as a system*. And I did. And when you create the correct system that accurately reflects what's actually happening, then it works. It works not just for that one thing that happened, it works for everything. And it doesn't involve leeches.

Teaching you to fish

The old adage says that if you teach someone to fish then they can feed themselves forever, as opposed to just handing them a fish. Fortunately the Sirens aren't handing you a fish. Oh no; they wouldn't do that. Instead they charge you a few hundred dollars for that fish. If you want more fish then just ask, and pay. And other kinds of fish? Well, that'll cost you too.

A *system* teaches you not only how to fish, but why that fishing works, so you can apply it to *other* fish.

Taking a step back

When people want to reach goals through the Alchemy for Life™ system, we don't just write down a bunch of goals. Instead we take two steps back, and fill out a colorful visual sheet online that shows where all their Time, Energy and Resources are going. Once we have that in place we then start to see a picture, and from that picture the goals spring forth. They are not random goals – they actually make sense. And since everything is mapped out we can actually make the time and the energy (and even reserve the resources) to make that goal happen. And you might even want a different goal than you initially thought you wanted.

Regardless of what or whom you pursue for your fish, make sure they are teaching you to fish instead of just selling you the fish.

Do you see how that is radically different than *their* formula:

You want to do X? I will help you do X and give me a lot of money.

Instead you will be taught to fish.

Regardless of what or whom you pursue for your fish, make sure they are teaching you to fish instead of just selling you the fish.

And keep your ship safe.

Mark Bradford

BALANCE COACHING

Now that you have a firm understanding of the Alchemy for Life™ concept (and hopefully you agree with it) allow me to detail what it is like to get coached with this method. Your curiosity, if any, can probably be summed up in four words:

"What do I get?" you ask.

I would preface my answer with - I like tangible stuff. Have I mentioned that already?

Tangible Stuff

When I read self-help books - or other non-fiction - I often scratch my head at the fact that I read that whole book only to get one or two bullet items. "Really?" I think, then shake my head, then toss the book into the bon fire. No, just kidding on the last thing.

When I meet other business professionals, or read posts on a site like LinkedIn, my eyes glaze over when they talk about synergy or other multi-syllable words that in real life mean very little. I'm a tangible guy (no that's not a comment about my fitness level - I think). I like tangible stuff, wrapping my arms around it, "getting it." You've probably encountered that word for the ninth[22] time in this book by now.

I'm betting most people like tangible stuff too. I'm betting you do too. So, you ask what's in this balance coaching for you? You wonder, what would actually happen if you did it? You don't need touchy feely stuff necessarily, you don't want a general "feeling." You want some sort of tangible result, an outcome, something that motivates you to do this.

Why can't I just tell you what you get, you may ask?

Well, unlike some of the other books out there, I can. And I want to.

What you get

You get more to work with. As I've said, balance coaching helps you to not only figure out your goals, but recover Time, Energy and Resources that you lost/are overspending along the way. This means you get more time to work with. That means you get more energy to use. That means you will have more resources to spend.

More time to use means you now have openings in a schedule that had no openings - or openings that are much larger, or planned, or lined up in a way that you're not scrambling from commitment A to commitment B.

More energy means you now have enough energy to work on that project - or hobby - that you dropped by the wayside. That means you get to do more of the thing you want to do, or just actually start doing the thing you have never been able to do.

---

[22] Thanks to Jonathan Pritchard, who lives in the future, for informing me that it's actually the *23rd* time.

More resources means you have more money, or more car time, or the availability of transportation that you didn't have before.

Actual Examples

Want examples? Sure. Here are specific examples partially taken from client results. They may not apply to you, but they are very real, very tangible results. So when you ask what you get, these are the things:

- You can now go out with your friends to wind down once a week, guilt free.
- Your wife now is actually interested in a date night - if you're wondering how your spouse would be affected by your balance, they are. In this case your wife has the energy and interest in date night, because you are now playing a greater role in being a parent, giving her more energy. Yes, your imbalance affects hers[23].
- You are now playing volleyball with friends again, and they are no longer nagging you.
- You are writing that book again, and you feel pretty good about it - you have a plan, a goal, and the time to do it.
- You're saving money on gas because you no longer have to drive your daughter to practice, and you have the car available to grocery shop, which means you're saving more money by not going out as much which also means you and your daughter are closer because you cook together every Wednesday and because you're closer and she feels more involved and takes ownership of chores. (there's actually more to this run on sentence! But, that's enough) See my post on the Sliding Puzzle for more on how so many things are connected.
- You don't hate your job, because you got a different one. After identifying that it was a huge imbalance and was draining all your energy you were able to get a new one.

---

[23] This could and should be an entirely separate discussion or book, don't you think?

We defined what you wanted, and why you weren't having any luck.

- You met a nice guy. You were about to give up on online dating, but we worked together, rewrote your profile and I explained some of the formula of how online dating works. You put in a fraction of the energy and got much better results.

- You are much healthier and lost some weight. All this time you enjoyed cooking, and just signing up for that healthy cooking class gave you more energy because you combined a passion with health. You got more energy twice: once for doing something you love, and once again because you're healthier doing it.

- You started a book club because you needed the socialization, and really didn't have a hobby. You didn't think "reading" was a hobby, but we made it both. Now you love reading even more and are considering writing.

- You see your parents more. You couldn't before because your schedule just didn't allow it, and you had that stress and guilt. I taught you how to shift things to open up your schedule, to prioritize the things you want to do. They really like the weekly visit. You don't have the guilt. You don't have that particular stress anymore.

- Your son is doing better in school because he has a tutor. The tutor cost minimal resources, and recovered time and energy. You thought it was too expensive, and felt it should be something you should be able to do. We figured out that it cost more *not* to have one, and that it reflected positively on your parenting to have one. You now have more time to work on other items while he is getting the help he needs, and you no longer feel guilty about him struggling.

- You found a church to go to like you've been wanting to do. But, until now you didn't have much direction and it was sort of daunting, especially with motivating the kids. Now that they are motivated by breakfast and stories afterwards they happily (for the most part) go.

Do any of these things sound like something you want? I could easily go on.

Stress-Free Productivity.

Imagine that: more productivity, less stress, at the same time. That's what balance coaching is - it's how you get to stress-free productivity. Perhaps "Stress-Free Productivity" coaching may not be as fluid as "Balance Coaching," but it tells you exactly what you get.

I know what you're going to say... "That's impossible! You don't understand my schedule, or how things work for me. That's like a Unicorn!"

Read on. It's not impossible.

Stressful vs. Stress-free

We all know what stress is. We all know (or hope we know) what productivity is. They typically go hand-in-hand. After all, the more effort you put into something the more you get out. Right? But if you want a few things (we all do) and not just one thing, you may find that more effort (Energy) in one creates a lack of effort in another. Same goes for Time and Resources. They fight each other. So you strive to find... balance. But even in finding balance you're making concessions and giving in and giving up in ways you may not like.

That pulling creates stress.

You may then switch to a denial mode in which you just keep pushing in both directions (sometimes it's three or more directions). You push and create stress and more stress until something gives. That something can be one of your tasks (sorry, I don't have time to meet up any more) health (high blood pressure from work), sanity (no fun, or overcompensation with adult beverages or substances) or even a relationship (you work too

73

much, we never have time for date night, you're always stressed from work).

That's *stressful* productivity. And that's life for most people - in varying degrees.

Stress-free Productivity is Feng shui and Fun

Stress-free productivity is not impossible. Not only that; it's actually more natural, more feng shui-like and more fun. By entering things on the Balance Sheet we can take a good look and map how you are currently doing things. We can then add what you'd like to do. Then we can work together, manipulate, test, discover and change. Then we map out how you'd like to do things. And then we do that. We do it with the Alchemy for Life™ system - a system complete with a supporting web application (Balance Sheet, Goals, Journal, Video).

And the unicorn appears. You can even pet him.

Mark Bradford

THE FORMULAS

This book is my way of helping you without helping you in person. If you read this and want to work with me - fantastic. In the mean time the following chapters are going to explain a number of ways you can get more control of your personal Alchemy for Life™ and get concocting some formulas. This is the good stuff; the self-help of the self-help book. This is the part people will probably flip to without reading the previous concepts and the whole point of "alchemy." Hopefully you *did* read that, because here's where we can have some fun.

Alchemical tomes[24]

Ancient books described various formulas the alchemists could follow to do various things with metals, herbs and health. Their formulas are fascinating to read through - albeit a bit hard to understand.

Our treatment of Time, Energy and Resources, and our spending those elements of life on the five established facets is an awful lot like the formulae of olde, isn't it? We visualize the flask filled (hopefully) with these mysterious and precious liquids. So why

---

[24] That's "tomes" and not "tombs." The latter refers to burial places; the former to ancient books.

not continue the fun of this metaphor? What would you call it when you figure out ways to combine this stuff in beneficial ways? Why alchemical formulas of course!

For example:

"I want my wife to have more energy for date night."

It is not:

"Just have her spend more energy on going on date night with you."

Why? Because the reality is she doesn't *have* the energy, because it's all tied up in parenting. So even if you solve the time issue, there's still the emotional gas that needs to be returned.

So the formula is:

You spend more energy co-parenting, which means you adjust your schedule so you can get the kids to the games, and free her up from some of those taxing responsibilities. But to do that you have to work smarter and have more time. You do that by working from home one day a week, and that makes you much more efficient and allows you the time to help out. The simple action of doing that inspires her and helps fill her emotional tank because you put effort into seeing her more.

Complicated, no?

Do you see how attempting to affect the energy and behavior of one person in a relationship actually requires you to adjust the other person?

That's why this "balance coaching" is done on a very visual system with notes and milestones.

That's why this kind of change typically requires some interaction.

But we can discuss some really good ways to understand the system. We will call them "formulas" but they are really chapters on very useful things you can do.

Formulas you can use

What you just read what quite a bit of overhead. You could call it a primer to coaching. By now you have a good grounding in what coaching is supposed to be, what it absolutely should not be, and the unique system I created to address it. You may even be curious about the latter.

Coaching yourself is comparable to being your own spotter at a gym. You're only one person, so you can't see yourself from another angle, another perspective. And, if your arms get weak you yourself cannot just grab the bar and help - thus averting a potentially dangerous outcome. Working out alone with weights to the point of fatigue should never be done alone like that.

Is coaching as useful and helpful as that? I hope you see that it is, when done properly. So I would not suggest you "coach" yourself.

However, I really want you to have all the tools moving forward. Just understanding coaching isn't enough. We have to understand what you encounter when you go out in the world and try to accomplish these goals - goals that I assume you had in mind when you picked up this book.

It's something I did a while ago and has helped so much I forgot I did it.

The second half of this book contains information you can use to navigate the road to completing your goals.

You'll find there is very little cheerleading even though what I will tell you may make you feel pretty darn good about getting that thing done.

If we consider all this to be alchemy, then imagine that the second half of this book are your magic formulas.

We will do the simplest thing we can to do get things going - we'll **start with Sunday**, for just **ten minutes**.

Then we will talk about a buzzword that wastes an awful lot of time and energy - **multitasking**. Understanding what it's not and how to use it properly will give you more time and energy to focus on what you want and bring you that much closer to your goals.

Then we will address **gaming the system**. Meaning, we can understand that the rules you think are in place are flawed, and no one is stopping you from bending them a bit.

I don't know what your goals are, but I hope this book helps you understand them, reach them and not beat yourself up on the way.

I'll introduce you to **an acronym** that will help you to get through the stuff that you don't want to do, by making an anchor with it. It's something I did a while ago and has helped so much I forgot I did it.

Do you have a comfort zone? Of course you do. You've heard people yell at you to move out of it. We'll talk about how it also may not be what you think, and some people who say they've moved outside of it haven't. You may **feel better about your comfort zone** after reading this.

An **understanding of time**, and how our perception changes the flow of it is very important to have. We'll get that, and you may be surprised that time can actually go slow when we are having fun -

it doesn't have to "fly."

Life has ups and downs, but we don't always consider that when reaching a goal; we seem to just program ourselves to succeed without any regard.

You've heard that you want to maintain your momentum, but does anyone ever talk about *the inertia of things in your life?* We will. Some things are easier to get started (or stop) than others. That consideration will help.

Different personalities require a different approach sometimes, and we will find out if *you value order over chaos.*

We will talk about *something that can affect the pursuit of any goal* - a part of your life that probably takes the most amount of energy and time from you - *your job.*

When you get close to your goal and things seem to *get harder*, we'll explain why by comparing it to pouring a beer or charging a battery.

Everyone has dread and doubt about decisions in their lives, even interaction with other people. That's normal, but if it's getting in the way of things we'll find out *what you can do in a day that dissolves both dread and doubt*.

Finally, we will talk about *being in the zone* and just how powerful that can be for you, whether you're there as part of seeking a goal or just doing what you love.

And after all that you won't be left on your own, you will be able to listen to the podcast every Sunday.

I don't know what your goals are, but I hope this book helps you understand them, reach them and not beat yourself up on the way.

START WITH SUNDAY

First and foremost we have to examine where you are in life. There's a way to do that in only ten minutes. People consider Sunday to be the off day, the Day of Rest, the day they tie up loose ends and wind up or down for the coming work week. If you work Sundays or have a non-traditional work week, then just replace Sunday with whatever day is technically your "Sunday." If you don't get a Sunday in any sense of the word, then STOP – we need to talk! You deserve a day of rest, you deserve a day in which you exert control over your Time, Energy and Resources. In fact, every day can and should be that way for you.

Sunday, however, is your day to catch up in case the week got out of control. Why not Saturday? Because Saturday is seen by many as the party day. Its seen as the *stay out late because there's still one more day* day. It's ingrained in popular American belief that Sunday is that day of rest, so use it to your advantage.

Even if your kids have a bunch of sports events to go to you can still exert your influence and take advantage of Sunday, and get some balance back. This includes getting balance in the coming week. Remember: planning is and continues to be your pal.

Find your place

First and foremost, you need to find a place - physical or mental - that allows you to do this magic. You can't do this reading the paper, or the iPad, or scrolling through Twitter. You can't do this "on-and-off" throughout the day. Maybe you can do this while cutting the grass, or in the car on the way to your friend, but let's not, OK? Find a place, get some mental, emotional and physical space between you and anything that needs your attention.

Use it as a look back. Think about this past week. Did you feel pulled apart? Was it a whirlwind? Did it move fast, or did it drag on? If it moved fast was that because your were busy doing really fun, fulfilling things, or because you were so overwhelmed in your job, or the combination of job and responsibilities you have at home?

Was there something you feel you really missed out on? Is there an "I wish I could have..." thought lingering? Is something nagging you that you could have done that you're going to carry into this next week? If so, that kind of baggage is just going to add stress.

Was there something that made it The Week From Hell? Was it a person, a boss? Was it a special week at work that screws up everything because everyone is stressed so because everyone is stressed everyone is stressed? Was it because a number of responsibilities all fell out of the sky at once and lined up to be The Perfect Crap-storm?

Find a place, get some mental, emotional and physical space between you and anything that needs your attention.

Is there something particularly great about this last week? If so, what was it? Was it a complete feeling because you got to do more varied (balanced) activities? Was it that a certain person or activity left you the hell alone this time? Was it simply that you *avoided* a stressful person, activity, etc? Was it something that you got to do that you never do – a chance to step up at work, fill in for your boss, lend a hand on a project? Did you get a chance to cook and make dinner because your partner was indisposed? Was your daughter's game cancelled and you got to just stay home and read that book?

Think about it. Think about it long and hard and explore, with your emotional memory, what it felt like. Then see the week for what it was.

Regardless of your answers here, just reviewing this allows you to learn from this. You may encounter a repeating pattern that once you see it you'll wonder why you didn't just fix it. And that's just as important for the good stuff too. You had that joy, do it again. That's what the balance coaching is about – figuring this stuff out with you, and then having foresight and fixing it, adjusting, squashing the bad, moving forward.

It's so simple but you don't do it.

So, do it.

Commit to do this on the next Sunday, regardless of it being six days from now or even if Sunday is today.

Think about it. Think about it long and hard and explore, with your emotional memory, what it felt like. Then see the week for what it was.

You may find it more helpful to do this at night as sort of a wind-down instead of doing it while you are staring at your yard while drinking a cup of coffee - whatever works for you to get these reflective, deceptively easy ten minutes to do this.

Formula for a better week:

Spend ten minutes reviewing what was painful, and what you really liked about last week. Then do your best to repeat the good stuff, and change/avoid the bad stuff.

So simple it sounds dumb, but no one really does this.

You will, now.

MULTITASKING AND THE FORGOTTEN GLUE

There's a huge myth regarding multitasking. Many believe multitasking is a near-magical ability to get more done; they believe that they have the ability to do two or more things at once – thus cheating the system. It makes anyone who can do this more valuable - perhaps even more important - they believe. Surely anyone in management, in high pressure positions, top performers – all of these are intense multitaskers performing two, three even four things _at the same time_.

The truth is that each time you have to switch gears from one task to another you expend energy. Mentally and or emotionally switching gears has a cost. That energy adds up, and can and will subtract from the energy available to perform the actual tasks. In most cases it also adds time.

Imagine a multitasker delivering a pizza, convinced at their ability to be master of time and space. They are to deliver the pizza and they decide to text their spouse about arranging a party. They discuss the planning, and the date and the guests. It's a lot of back and forth and since they don't want to die and are unsure of the location, they only text while stopped. Because of this they get beeped at by a driver behind them more than once, as they were trying to finish a sentence at a stoplight and it has turned green. Then they get beeped at again. *Just let me finish this, oh fine.* They drive off, but are thinking about the point they were trying to make. They miss a turn, but it's not a big deal because they can just take the next one.

The truth is that each time you have to switch gears from one task to another you expend energy.

They get to the destination and finally they have the time to finish this conversation. Just a few back-and-forths, and we can run the pizza up to the house. Conversation has mostly ended, though there are a few things but they better get this pizza out. They do, and it's cold. They lost track of time trying to do both, and the conversation ended up being sort of convoluted and not clear, since she rushed more than once with all the impatient drivers behind her.

Notice how I didn't combine driving with a simple phone call. I am talking about combining *two meaningful tasks that require true attention.* And I didn't want anyone to crash. Obviously, a part of Alchemy for Life™ is about a form of overlap that could be considered multitasking. It is applied carefully when the two items are *using the same kind of thought patterns*, or it combines *a major task with a lesser "autopilot" task.* Examples of this are folding laundry while watching guilty pleasure TV, dusting while on a conference call, learning a new skill by reading a book while waiting for your daughter at an event. These items do not include texting while driving, helping your son with homework while reading an email, or having an intense discussion about your relationship while doing your taxes. Folly, pure folly I say unto you!

Alchemy includes course corrections

When you understand what Alchemy for Life is about, and you work in the Balance Sheet, you see that these course corrections are considered. You find that energy is returned that you didn't think was being expended. Also, it's not just the time being spent on a task you reduce or remove, it's also the energy *between* the tasks. It's the glue holding the multitasking together.

Next time you try to multitask, don't just consider the Time, Energy and Resources you think you might save, consider the glue holding the multitasking together. Picture yourself pouring some of your flask's liquid into task number one, then some into task number two *AND a little to maintain them both at the same time*. Like a tax, or a cost of doing business - or a glue holding it all together. If you don't have enough energy to afford that, or you choose two tasks that are not a good fit (two major tasks for example) it could cost you more than it's worth. Both tasks will be done poorly. If the point of multitasking for you is to be a mover and shaker that accomplishes a lot of excellent work, you'll end up doing the opposite.

> # Next time you try to multitask, don't just consider the Time, Energy and Resources you think you might save, consider the glue holding the multitasking together.

Consider the glue. Consider the kind of tasks you are combining. Then consider moving and/or shaking.

And a last note: working on a task while you are waiting for something isn't really "multitasking." So if you think you are an awesome multitasker who can do two major tasks but one of the tasks is just waiting for an email, or a phone call then you are in reality just doing one task while you wait for another.

If you'd like to move and/or shake at the same time that you do a bunch of other things, consider the above.

Formula for multitasking properly:

Combine only one major task with a lesser autopilot task.

THE FLAW IN THE SYSTEM

I was chatting with a friend recently. He is constantly flying around the US selling the services of his firm. He relayed to me that he - unlike most people trying to do the same thing - had found the flaw in the system. The system he was referring to was the selling of fungible services to extremely sophisticated clientele. His understanding of the flaw in the system and ability to exploit it gives him a massive advantage over the many others doing the same thing. He wins - over and over again.

Game Mechanics

It reminded me of the olden days, way back when I ran a small game company. I was always fascinated with game theory and game mechanics, and spent many hours dissecting board games, card games[25], and games in general. After a while I could see the patterns, and ultimately the flaws. The best games had few flaws, but they all had 'em. Some had obscenely obvious flaws - games like Monopoly, that made Grandma throw the board at you after a few hours of playing, for example. If you figured out the flaw in a

---

[25] I recently came out with a card game that simulated relationships.

game you could exploit it, and win - over and over again. Sorry Grandma.

My job in creating a game was to create playable fun rules that had as few exploitable flaws as possible. The rules that were there seemed logical and fair. It was fun, and I created two RPGs and two card games.

There's an order to things. Is there though?

Life is a game. It has rules, playing pieces and all that stuff. The more you play it, the better you get. I'm not talking about reincarnation[26], that'd be an entirely different kind of book. I'm talking about the accumulated wisdom, and the understanding of things that are either invisible or extremely subtle to the average person - the seeing of patterns and flaws.

The flaw in the system

So, what's the flaw in that system? Life has some pretty hard and fast rules. You have to have a job, you have to work a certain amount, money is prevalent in everything you do. Most people are investing in a relationship, you have to eat right or pay the consequences, etc. Right?

Games like Monopoly, that made Grandma throw the board at you after a few hours of playing, for example.

You have to work every day, eight plus hours. Do you though?

You have to put a certain amount of time in things to get a desired

---

[26] I already wrote a book on that - *OneSelf: Have faith. In yourself.*

result. Do you though?

You have to do things a certain way like everyone else does. Do you though?

There's an order to things. Is there though?

The manual

First of all, life doesn't exactly come with a manual. Sure there are those that will argue with me and cite certain ancient texts or books. I'm not talking about how you should live your life, I'm talking about the mechanics of existence. Understanding the mechanics and the options you have that you weren't even aware of gives you a massive advantage over those that don't. You win. Again and again.

The score

In life we keep score usually by tracking a few things - wealth, friends, stuff, happiness, status[27]. How are you keeping score? Are you comparing your happiness to others? Are you comparing your status in the company you're in to a coworker's? Do you have the same vacation, parachute, benefit package, upward mobility? Are you comparing your house to the Jones' across the street?

Time Energy and Resources

You know I can't write a chapter without mentioning Time, Energy and Resources. Life is made of those three things - you hear me say - over and over again. It's because it's true. Everything we do is made up of one or more of those - either giving or receiving.

---

[27] Status is a common theme in relationships, and something I talk about extensively. See www.thestatusgame.com for more info on that subject.

The board

Some games have a board, and they are usually referred to as board games (for obvious reasons). The board is a nice visualization; it helps you to see where you are, if you're winning, how close you are to your goal.

Along with not being given a manual for life, you are also not given a board. Sure you may have a calendar to help you track time, or to do lists to help you track activities, but you can't really see how you're doing overall. You can't see how you are doing as compared to your potential, and you can't see how one thing affects the other. There's very little journaling and the journalling you may do is in general.

The Balance Sheet

That's why I invented the balance sheet. It's a way to see all of the aforementioned things. That's why I created the unified journaling that ties the journaling to the activities and the goals. It's really cool and you should see it. So, using this balance sheet we exploit some of the flaws in the system - for your benefit[28].

Here is an example of one the mechanics of life, and how we can exploit it.

Time is linear, activities are not

Unless you are an extra-dimensional being, or enlightened in ways we can't even describe here, time is linear for you[29]. That means that time goes in a straight line from before to now to what happens next. However, activities do not have to be linear. If you have two activities you participate in, it is possible to combine them, to stack them, to blend them in such a way so that they are occurring at the same time. Instead of being lined up, one in front

---

[28] You're going to experience some of this with the worksheets at the end of the book.

[29] Listen to my podcast, "Why are you here."

of the other, they are being stacked on top of each other.

Multitasking is the big lie, the misleading productivity thing that everyone brags about, nobody actually does and in the end makes you less productive.

That's just multitasking you say? No, it's not. Multitasking is the big lie, the misleading productivity thing that everyone brags about, nobody actually does and in the end makes you less productive. Check out the various studies, like the one done in 2008 University of Utah, or the fun little read on the network structure of our brain. No, I'm not talking about multitasking.

Will it blend?

I'm talking about taking a step above your timeline and administratively blending two activities together. Huh? What did those words mean? They meant, from a coaching position, and being your Temporal Spotter, that I would review the balance sheet and blend two activities together that are of the same tone, that don't require you to switch brain networks. You know what I'm talking about - when you do find two things that are kind of fun to do together, like emptying the dishwasher and chatting on the phone. Like reading fiction on the elliptical. I'm not talking about responding to emails while having a conversation, or texting and driving.

So, blend two activities that can use the same brain network, that you want to do (or don't want to do) and cheat and get more time back. Trust me, there are things you're doing right now that can be blended. And, not only will you not lose anything about the experience, you may actually enjoy both more. Or, you'll dislike one less once it becomes blended. This works particularly well with teens.

I can tell you that I programmed my brain to get up and do housework when I get a social call. I have a successful friend that calls me all the time, and my son calls from Germany via FaceTime audio.
I got so used to this habit of doing housework via phone call that one day I went to empty the dishwasher and it was already emptied. "Who the hell emptied the dishwasher already?" I thought. I didn't remember doing it. My autopilot did it. I enjoyed both the phone call and the housework more.

Think about that. I got to catch up with my son, and get some mundane house work done - pretty much automatically. You may think this is not a big deal, but little things like that add up, especially when they start to happen automatically.

See the next chapter for much more detail on this, and the rest of the book for more flaws to exploit.

<u>Formula for exploiting the flaws in the system:</u>

Make your own board since there is none. Track and see your progress in a way that others cannot, combine things you normally wouldn't.

DO IT TO A F.A.U.L.T.

That's a fun acronym. I created this acronym to help you and me remember what those words stand for. And it worked, because I quickly forgot about the concept, until I remembered the acronym.

Ever heard that someone does something "to a fault?" I won't get into how that phrase is abused and how it's essentially used as a virtue signal, but it does conjure up a certain image in our mind doesn't it?

When someone does something *to a fault* you are to believe that they do it pretty much no matter what, right? They are so committed to it that you can count on them for that particular attribute. So doing something to a F.A.U.L.T. is very similar.

In previous chapters we talked about a special kind of blending of tasks. Yes you can call it multitasking, but it's really the best kind of "multitasking."

As I said most people look at multitasking as the ability to handle a number of requests at a time and juggle them. My position (and it is backed by the two aforementioned studies) is that this kind of multitasking is counter-productive, uses a lot of energy, is stressful and really not what people think it is.

So instead I'm talking about that blending of activities that require the same sort of thought patterns. But we already discussed that, so what is this F.A.U.L.T. thing about?

F.A.U.L.T. stands for Feeling, Activity, Unconditionally, Location, or Time.

Remember the emptying of the dishwasher when I got a social call? If I received a social call when I was working (or not) and had the energy to talk (maybe I was in the middle of work, or feeling introverted), I would immediately stop what I was doing and do some housework as long as I was talking.

I wanted to empty the dishwasher but thought for a split second, "I wish my son would call so I could have clean forks."

It was automatic. In fact so automatic that I couldn't figure out who the hell snuck in my house and emptied the dishwasher. How did this happen? Because I did it to a F.A.U.L.T.

Feelings

You can do the same with feelings. It's a well known psychological lever to connect something to a feeling, and in some cases is even more powerful to disconnect them. You associate rock climbing with your ex-boyfriend so now you don't enjoy it. That's unfortunate. Rock climbing is a good activity, and was always enjoyable. Now your brain connects the feeling of loss and all the bad feelings of your break up with one of your favorite hobbies.

But what if the reverse is true? What if you met a great guy at rock climbing. You dated for a bit and then he moved away for work (you knew it was going to happen while you were dating and you both just enjoyed the time you had). So in that case you continue to be motivated to rock climb because you have good feelings associated with it. Maybe you'll never meet another guy because of it, but even when you feel a little tired something in you just says that some handsome man might be there.

If you went to church as a child you may remember a promise of ice cream afterwards, or some snack in church if you were quiet.

You didn't look forward to the snack or the ice cream. You looked forward to the *feeling* those things provided. Your parent helped connect the feeling of having ice cream with going to church. And in the case of the snacks it was a blending because they happened at the same time.

They combined the uncomfortable/unpleasant[30] experience of church with the pleasant feeling of snacking. It tasted good and made you feel special, and made you feel liked by your parents because you were behaving.

Our brain unfortunately makes all sorts of emotional connections to things without our participation. We know that, advertisers know that, psychologists know that, NLP practitioners know that, people who treat trauma such as PTSDs all know that.

So why not use this ability to your advantage? Why not also connect a pleasant feeling with an activity you want to do or should do?

Want other examples?

"No pain, no gain." How many people associate a good feeling with working out? When you get into working out and want to stick with it you have to eventually do some sort of mental manipulation or you're just not going to finish it. As I've said we

---

[30] From the perspective of a young child.

are not robots, and our physical energy is not what prevents us from working out - it's the emotional gas. If you can add to the tank while working out, or just when thinking about it you are much more likely to follow through.

If you associate cleaning with having control over your environment, I can bet you that if you have a day in which you thought you were losing control, you found a way to clean your bathroom, or your bedroom for "no reason."

So use this to your advantage.

Activities

It's a powerful thing to blend activities - especially as I said the blending of one you don't like with one you do. All my brain remembers is the fun chat with my son, not the housework. How did I get that to the point that I'm pretty much incapable of just laying on the couch chatting? Because of the "A" in F.A.U.L.T.: *Activity.* I assigned the task of having a pleasant phone call to the activity of getting up and doing housework.

You can do the same with two activities. You probably already do. A lot of people connect driving with listening to an audiobook. It becomes so ingrained that they scramble to find other audiobooks when it looks like they are running out. In fact you can imagine that this can go a little too far, humorously. It did for me. I wanted to empty the dishwasher but thought for a split second, "I wish my son would call so I could have clean forks."

Imagine someone saying, "I'd love to drive over but I don't have any audiobooks." Huh?

Unconditionally

OK, so this one was shoved in here because as much as I loved F.A.L.T. I thought there must be a "U" lurking out there that makes sense. It's the odd man out as it's not exactly anchored in the way the others are. If you can't find a reasonable anchor for your task, you may just end up resolving to do it no matter what - that's what "unconditionally" means. This is the physiological method some people have to resort to when they make life changing decisions and quit drinking or smoking cold turkey. It's sort of like throwing a switch in your mind - click - *I'm doing this, period.*

Location

I have a nice quiet office in my home, two giant monitors, all the software I need, privacy and the ability to listen to any music I want on demand. Also there's a refrigerator filled with food. The coffee maker serves coffee inexpensively. I can work in my pajamas if I want.

But what do I do? I go to a cafe with a MacBook air, which has a smaller screen. I bring my headphones to block out the sound, I buy coffee at three times the cost I get it for at the store, the food available is also much more expensive and far more limited. It costs Time, Energy and Resources just to drive there and back. And, as people now recognize me, there is a very real chance of being interrupted for an extended period of time as they sit down and chat.

Why? Am I crazy? Well, maybe, but that's another book. No, it's because I attached the act of digging deep in writing to a *location*. And that location is not my office[31]. Unless you are a real estate mogul, you don't have unlimited properties to choose from, but instead choose public venues and have to deal with the ups and downs of that location.

You can be like me and ignore a perfectly good environment for one that is less convenient, more costly, more variable and requires more effort to get to. But then, this is my fourth book, thanks in

[31] Paradoxically I wrote this paragraph in my office. This was because i had to print some things before I wrote this. Go figure.

part to this inefficient and illogical psychological anchoring.

It works. I like it, I look forward to being "rewarded" with "cafe time" and my writing time feels more legitimate.

You can and should do the same thing.

Time

Probably the easiest to understand, as most of us use this to get through life. Does your brain still wake you up on the weekend at 6:00am? That's because you associate 6:00am with getting up for work. You wake up on Saturday at 6:00am, look at the clock, then realize you can stay in bed. If you are a normal person you say "Whoo hoo" and go back to sleep. I get up, but that's my personal problem.

If you have a task you want to get done, you can attach it to a time. This may seem really obvious but it is not, because there are lots of tasks that we simply never do that with. And, even more powerfully, you can make this kind of attachment with a block of time with an *intention*. What do I mean by that?

Writing every day - writing to a F.A.U.L.T.

Because of my schedule and my desire to write, a long time ago I assigned 7:00am-8:00am as "writing time." That means from 7-8 I have to write something. The rule for that block of time is that the writing has to be creative - whether it is an article, part of a story, part of a book, or something else. It has to be creative, it cannot be an email and it cannot be "work related."

So though I am not connecting a task, I am connecting an intention (with rules) to that hour of time. I don't always have that block of time to write, but I usually do.

What could you accomplish if you assigned Saturday morning

from 9:00am-10:00am for housework? Maybe you already do that. But if you don't you would be surprised at how much you can get done in only an hour. And if your family knows this and you stick to it, you will find that something amazing happens: *they will start to adjust their schedules to yours.* Your family and friends will "get" that Saturday morning for that hour is cleaning time. Your kids will be less likely to resist your requests for help because they no longer resent you, they see it as calendar item and they'll find it difficult to resent a calendar.

The point of the F.A.U.L.T. acronym is to remind you that you can use these psychological hooks to anchor something so that you do it on an ongoing basis and accomplish something. Accomplishing something based on an anchor like this is very likely, almost inevitable.

It works. I like it, I look forward to being "rewarded" with "cafe time" and my writing time feels more legitimate.

You may not like cleaning your house, but if you know it makes you (F)eel like you have control you're more likely to do it - especially when the negative feeling of losing control creeps in.

If you are just going to get housework done whenever, it's less likely to get done than if it is anchored to another pleasurable (A)ctivity (social phone calls).

You might be at your wit's end so you decide to (U)nconditionally do something because things have gotten that serious (in your mind at least and that's all that matters).

You may think you want to find a way to write a book, but you're more likely to get in all the hard, meaty, time-consuming work if you assign it to a public (L)ocation like a cafe.

You may say you're going to work out more, but you're probably going to get it done if you know it happens at a specific (T)ime on Tuesdays and Thursdays.

It is important to note that all this would be seen as being part of NLP (Neuro-Linguistic Programming). In my humble opinion it is not. Why? Because NLP is the latest buzzword for anything remotely psychological. By placing the NLP label on this I feel that it disconnects it from everything else in this book as a whole.

Call it what you want, of course. If you think it is NLP, then so be it. To me it is a fun acronym that represents the anchoring of tasks to one of five realities.

<u>Formula for accomplishing things you don't want to:</u>

Anchor tasks to Feelings, Activities, Unconditionally, Locations or Times.

COMFORT ZONES

Comfort Zones

You have heard lots of helpful phrases regarding your comfort zone. You've heard phrases like "Move out of your comfort zone" or "Nothing ever happens in the comfort zone" or "Make it a point to move out of your comfort zone on a regular basis" or "The Comfort zone is for loading and unloading of passengers only."

You've probably heard so many helpful phrases like that that you:

- Feel bad about actually having a comfort zone. How dare you?
- Have no interest in moving out of it, since the outside of it sounds cold, barren and uncharted.

I don't blame you. That's how I felt hearing about all that. In fact, talks about comfort zones is in the same category as "success" and "goals" for a lot of people - it's a place that most people don't go. It's not for them, it's only something professional athletes or people who have some sort of personality disorder - crazy go getters who are Type A always smiling with big teeth shaking hands and injuring arms. Meanwhile you're just working hard, paying the bills, making sure your clients and/or boss and/or spouse doesn't dislike you.

You are too busy working hard and doing all that stuff you do inside this demonized space called The Comfort Zone.

They can take they "success" and "goals" and keep 'em. You are too busy working hard and doing all that stuff you do inside this demonized space called The Comfort Zone.

Feh. Perhaps even Double Feh.

The Comfort Zone - what it actually is

The comfort zone is not a bad thing. We all have one. We all *need* one. Like love, creativity and desire, it's an illusive thing. The more you define it and become aware of it, the more it slips away, shifts and becomes undefinable. Some of that space exists based on how we are programmed with our DNA, other parts are due to upbringing and environment. Still more of it we create as we go along. It's part of life, and a necessity for mental health and... you guessed it, balance.

And, like all things, we can misuse it and things become out of balance.

The Dome

I live in a large town near a small town. I won't tell you the name except to say that it rhymes with "Omarosa." I have learned through the years that more often than not the good people who live there do not like to leave it. Surely they must leave it from time to time to visit other municipalities, go on vacation, go to work, etc. However, if you schedule a meeting with someone from there, they will almost invariably suggest the meeting takes place inside this small town. Mind you, this is not a small town that is like an oasis in the middle of the desert, separated from another oasis by a stretch of road through the dangerous dessert. No, it is just a section of a larger county; it has borders like any other municipality. If you drive through it you will not even have a clue you've passed into it, or driven through it - other than the "Welcome to ..." sign you might see.

But *they* know. Like occupants of a magical dome, they know when they've left the dome - and they do what they can to prevent that.

The meetings can be a beer with a friend, a date, or a business meeting. Every date I've had with someone from The Dome has occurred literally a block or two away from where the other person actually lives.

Why is this? I don't know. It's a nice place, with a tiny town center, but I haven't figured that out. Or perhaps I have. Perhaps the population of this small town all share a comfort zone more intensely than most, thus creating a magical, invisible barrier.

Yeah, let's go with that.

Why do I mention this?

Because it's a great, almost physical example of a comfort zone stretched too far.

The Comfort Zone, Goals and a Schedule

Now that we know having a Comfort Zone is not a bad thing, and we are not going to attack the fact that you not only have one but enjoy said zone, how do we work with it? My approach to coaching is always to look at the whole, and not just target one seemingly obvious culprit. We're much more interesting than that.

Here's what to be aware of and how to work with it.

Become aware of your Comfort Zone. Is it being around people? Is it always working on paper and not with people? Is it something as small and contained as just being snuggled on the couch in PJs watching trashy TV? Is it working with a certain age of people, eating a certain food, eating a lot of a certain foods, or eating a lot of a certain food very often?

Once you know you're in your comfort zone, you can think about how big it is.

Sometimes your Comfort Zone contributes to your success. Yes really. You don't hear that often, do you?

Take steps to move out of it, on a regular basis. Making it a point to do this will have a great impact on your successes - you'll have more, move faster towards your goals and have some surprises along the way. Why? Because like the good people of The Dome, the magical barrier prevents you from doing or even seeing something that would lead to success and happiness.

When we work together, we figure this out, and we figure out how your Comfort Zone affects what you want to do. Yes, sometimes, like the people in The Dome, it prevents you from doing something simple; it prevents you from making progress exploring options that other people take for granted. Sometimes your comfort zone contributes to your success. Yes really. You don't hear that often, do you?

A Comfort Zone is a matter of perspective

A Comfort Zone, again, is not a bad thing. Like anything else *too much of it* is a bad thing, but not enough is also a bad thing. If anyone - a business associate, a motivational speaker, anyone -

tells you that they are "always outside their comfort zone" they are a Big Fibbing Doo Doo Head[32]. What they've done is construct a career around an existing Comfort Zone, one that contains the elements that makes them happy and comfortable. But, because the space is kind of scary to the average person - speaking to crowds, selling, traveling, etc., they can sell it as being *outside* their zone. They are not.

A shark is perfectly comfortable in water, in the dark. Humans are perfectly comfortable surrounded by air in the light, on land. If a shark builds a career out of swimming in the dark, cold waters, he's not outside of his Comfort Zone.

He's outside of yours.

So when you think of Comfort Zones, do not feel bad about having one. If you stretch it too far, think of The Dome.

You will want to try out some of the things in this book if it makes you feel uncomfortable - because that's outside of your comfort zone.

Formula for additional and accelerated success:

- Figure out your Comfort Zone
- Take steps to move outside of it and see what happens
- Be aware of the discomfort and fear that you experience when moving outside of it
- Don't beat yourself up for enjoying your Comfort Zone - you deserve to have one

---

[32] Sorry for the language.

TIME COMPRESSION

I recently gave a talk to some very interested kids on writing fiction. One of the things I told them was that they had control over time. I explained that when writing a story - unless something interesting is happening, or important to the story - we typically jump over it. On the flip side of that is the ability to expand time when something very important is happening.

I told them that time moves faster when you are interested but when you are bored it seems to drag on. Demonstrating this, I said that if they found my talk boring they would be fidgeting, looking around, checking the clock and every time they'd look back at it the minute hand would have barely moved. If they paid attention and were in the moment, before they knew it it would be over.

For some reason they all sat up and paid attention.
In compressing time further I explained how we could spend pages just describing the ten seconds someone had in trying to catch an explosive that was about to go off. Those were important moments. It was all a matter of attention and perception. You define the important moments.

The same is true for productivity.

It will not surprise you that when you are enjoying a task time seems to go by quickly. It will also not surprise you that the opposite is true; that time drags on when something is not so desirable.

Here are two things that will probably surprise you about time and productivity.

Time can go slow for the things you do like.

Getting "lost" in our work is a good thing, but we sometimes push things to the limit when we are good at them, especially if you're a Type A Mover & Shaker. The first thing you think of when you read "increasing your productivity" is "doing more things in less time" right? We cram more and more into the same amount of time, until we feel rushed and have sucked all the life and fun out of it. It doesn't help when there are so many articles and tips on increasing your productivity. Present company excluded of course.

Productivity is efficiency, and efficiency is proper flow

What you, and most people forget is that productivity is also efficiency. The miles per gallon[33] your car is capable of is usually stated in City / Highway miles. Highway is always higher, why? Because traveling on the highway is done at higher speeds the engine was designed for, there is less stopping and starting and machines operate better when they can just go. Note that the engine will also become less efficient if you push it out of the efficient zone to, say, 160 mph. Not only a bad idea for your efficiency, but not a good idea for your safety, the safety of others, and those pesky court appearances once the cars with the flashing lights catch up to you. Also there's a film crew.

---

[33] Or "MPGe" for electric cars.

Efficiency is happiness

OK, ok. You see a long corridor of people dressed in spartan military outfits, pulling levers, and they're all shouting that - "Efficiency is happiness!" Some sort of sad violin music with no bass is playing from overhead speakers. No, that's not what I meant.

Your efficiency is tied to your happiness. When you are happy and in the flow, you're on the highway, speeding along, doing your thing. It feels right. It's your speed, man. Remember that time you did that thing you like at exactly the speed you were comfortable with? Yeah, that was awesome.

So having the proper efficiency, i.e. - going at the speed that feels best doing the thing you are good at - can really feel great.

Have you ever noticed that some really great businesses cease to exist when the expand and get into the big market? The cause is not just that their product creation doesn't scale. The failure is because the creation of items are very closely tied with the time and efficiency of the creator. When this efficiency is "increased" due to production methods the actual product (and enjoyment of the creator) changes as well.

Think about attempting to mass produce glass blowing. Sometimes a thing is meant to be done in small batches, with care and love and that's as "efficient" as that's going to get.

Formula for more efficiency and more happiness doing tasks:

- Find the speed at which you are happiest - it may be faster and it may be slower than you've been doing it[34]
- Be mindful and in the moment when you are doing a task as that will slow down enjoyable time
- Do not be persuaded by efficiency for the sake of efficiency

---

[34] With the understanding that this may affect others on your team, yes.

EVERYONE FINDS TIME...

"Everyone finds time for what they really want to do."
My friend recently repeated this phrase to me in response to a story
I told him. He finds perverse pleasure in doing that, since I coined
the phrase some time ago.   He likes to repeat it back to me, to use
it as a talisman, and to reference it as if some great philosopher
spoke it a thousand years ago.

My friend makes it clear that the concept is not something he
hadn't considered (he's pretty quick to monitor praise and also
makes sure he's not revealing a lack of knowledge), but rather that
it is spelled out so simply.

That's what people do – they find the time to do what they really
want. I'm not suggesting that we have complete control over every
moment, and at any second on a whim we just do what feels good.
However, we do have a lot more control than we let on. And
sometimes we have more control than we will admit, and then
comes the excuses.

Awareness is the first step

It becomes obvious once you are aware of it. When someone says
"I'd love to but I have to do blank instead" that's usually a flag.

People in sales know this, and have many ways to work around it. Most of these ways are not very effective, because the person in question just doesn't want to do it.

When you become aware that others do that it gives you a window into their priorities. It can also cause you to be a bit offended – "I'd love to see you but *I just washed my hair and can't do a thing with it.*"

The friend I mentioned? He was so tickled by this phrase that has taken it upon himself to call out some people on this. He found out, the hard way, that people do not like to be called out on this. Understandably, like many things that make up our psyche, it is part of a complex structure of protective layers. Like all things ingrained in you it is there for a reason. Sometimes the reason is silly, sometimes it's not. Usually it's protected by safety measures that can kick in when questioned.

I'm not at all suggesting that you question your friends, family and acquaintances every time they are not available – "What are you doing instead...? *AHA!*" Unless you want a lot less friends, family and acquaintances.

But that is where the fun begins. For my friend, it's the fun of seeing the look of recognition and uncomfortableness. For me it's the realization and "aha" moment they get – it's the moment I just handed the steering wheel back to them.

The workplace is different

We do this all the time in the workplace too; we find the time to do the things we want to do. That's when we assess what we are doing, and what we'd rather be doing. The difference is that in the workplace what we *want to do* is replaced by what we *are supposed to be doing*. In some cases those things are done in compliance with what fits with the mission statement, the culture and the job description. In other cases it is what is needed to get the job done effectively, and in other cases those are one in the same (mission, culture and job description define the things that get the job done effectively, productively and competitively). We give it labels like Time Management, Process Improvement and Prioritization.

In other cases, unfortunately, it truly is what the person *wants* to do – being on Facebook, surfing the web, streaming Netflix, shopping, handling personal business via endless calls and emails. Let's just assume that you're not one of these people and never speak of this again.

In our private lives we are much more territorial about this, and we develop protective justifications.

As I was saying, in business we accept what we are supposed to be doing - sometimes begrudgingly - but it is accepted nonetheless. We know that one thing is supposed to take priority over another, and often times we have a manager that will remind us of this. In fact, your job may be in part or in whole to keep others on track in this way, with you being the leader and effective coach of the team.

In our private lives we are much more territorial about this, and we develop protective justifications. In business we can't or aren't supposed to develop these justifications because this prioritization is part of the job. Of course that doesn't stop many from finding ways to still develop protective justifications for not doing what they are supposed to be doing. That's what gages the effectiveness of some employees – their ability to be doing just what they are "supposed to be doing" at any given moment. And that's what sometimes defines an employee who is not so effective – they tend to focus on the wrong things, in the wrong order, etc. Their manager has to spend a lot of time refocusing them on a task they *should* be doing instead of what they *are* doing.

Having the autonomy of working on just what you are supposed to is a valuable and underrated asset.

So what then?

<u>Formula for understanding how you and others handle time:</u>

- If you receive it as a reason, **you can now recognize it.** You now know what "I don't have time for that" really means

- **Don't give it as reason unless it's true and you actually want to do that thing**. Someone, like you, may be enlightened to this fact and you will end up being more transparent than you intended. Instead try the more direct route with them. And be honest with yourself. *Do I really not have time, or do I just not want to do it?*

- **If you are giving this reason** a lot **you are spending** a lot of **effort avoiding conflict**. In the end this is going to cause more effort and time than it's worth. It is a crutch that can worsen a weakness you already have.

- Comparing **what someone is *supposed to be doing* and what they *are doing* is a helpful measurement**. Arguably, the closer those things are to being one in the same, the better fit they are for a job or career. One can argue that they just need coaching, aren't right for the culture, etc. Regardless it's a simple gage, and very revealing.

LIFE'S UPS AND DOWNS

You've heard this before right? "Life has ups and downs." You're typically told this when something bad happens, or you encounter a challenge. If things are difficult with your kids then someone might tell you about the rollercoaster it is to have them. If you are having job difficulties, or are between jobs, or your relationship is on the rocks you'll be told about the ups and downs.

No one seems to do the reverse, even though it is perfectly accurate and valid.

If you tell someone that you just got a promotion, the response is never that life has "ups and downs." If you tell your bestie that you and Matt are really getting along and you think he's going to ask you to marry him next Saturday she doesn't remind you that you'll also have bad times!

That would be rude, right? Rude, accurate, perceptive and true.

As humans we like to focus on the good stuff. In fact, our memories are structured in such a way as to easily remember the good stuff. This is why you can have an up and down relationship with someone and then start missing them - even though they were a jerk. Your brain just highlights the fun stuff.

Is there anything wrong with this? No, it's normal. But like anything else, if overused it can be detrimental.

Any strength stretched too far becomes a weakness.

If you focus too much on the good stuff, and just forget about the bad, or ignore the fact that life has ups and downs, you will set yourself up for failure - more failure than you expected.

Paradoxically over-focusing on the positive can cause you to be ill-prepared and lack the resilience needed when you hit a snag.

That would be rude, right? Rude, accurate, perceptive and true.

The point of telling you this is so that you can navigate properly.

If you are going for a long drive - expecting it to be a straight line - but encounter a lot of curves, you may think you are going in the wrong direction. You might even give up.

If you do everything you can to give yourself and your family a good life but bad stuff happens you might take ownership of it, and beat yourself up. You might make changes you didn't need to make.

However, if you look at a map before your drive and expect these turns - the construction, the possibility of needing to take an alternate route - you'll measure the success of the trip differently.

If something happens with your family that you know is out of your control and part of life then you will just be supportive, and make it through together, instead of taking it upon your shoulders for no reason.

Ups and downs.

Ups and downs and goals

The reason this made it into this book is to prepare and explain to you that since it's a part of life, it's a part of goals. If you keep your eyes open and look at the map[35], or you know that not every day is progress but instead learning from mistakes, you are much more likely to reach your goal. And, you'll become a better person along the way.

This is why some people give up - because their internal, pristine, fanatical version of success doesn't match what is happening in real life. So, they decide to stop.

Don't stop, be realistic and understand that life has ups and downs.

<u>Formula for navigating ups and downs:</u>

- Recognize that there are both ups and downs
- When in a down remember that there are ups, and take strength from that
- When it an up, remember that there are downs and cherish that moment more
- Do not create a fantastical expectation, thus creating a false down
- Remember that so many things in life are cyclical

---

[35] In my case, the balance sheet. :)

INERTIA AND MOMENTUM

Let's be real

Let's be real.   You know, like totally real here. No, I'm not going to reveal an inner secret, I do that enough indirectly in my podcasts already. Also, you read the "My Story" chapter and had enough probably. No, I mean let's discuss the physical world.

We've all heard about inertia and momentum, but few people know the difference. Sure, metaphorically people say "I'm building momentum" but even fewer ever say anything about their inertia.

What? Right.

So, stay real with me here and then we can go metaphorical...
 Inertia is derived from the Latin word "iners", which means *idle* or *lazy*. Interesting, eh? Inertia is a measurement of *how lazy the system is*. Literally. It's literally described as being a measurement of "how lazy a system is." See where I'm going yet?

An object at rest stays at rest and an object in motion stays in motion with the same speed and in the same direction unless acted upon by an unbalanced force. Meaning, if something is just sitting there, that's what it's going to do. If something is moving, that's what it's going to keep doing, unless something messes with it.

Rocks and Feathers

A big rock is just going to sit there. A feather is not, even though they are both sitting there. Why does the feather move? Because it is affected by the external forces easier than the big rock. They are both being pulled upon by gravity, both being randomly pelted by rain, sleet or what we like to call precipitation in Wisconsin: a "wintry mix." And they both are being accosted by wind. Aha. Because of the lightness of the feather it is less anchored. Because of the surface of the feather, it is subjected to catching the wind.

If you take a picture of a big rock, you can't tell if it's a still day, or the middle of a hurricane unless there's visible precipitation. However, on a still day the feather lays there, on a windy day it's zooming around and now it's not in the picture anymore.

A baseball thrown in space at 80 miles an hour is going to keep going through space for a very very long time, at 80 miles an hour. Nothing is messing with it - not air resistance, not gravity, nothing. Sure there are particles it's going to hit, and microgravity from everything in the universe - a nearby star or planet or moon, but noticeably it just keeps going. Throw that same baseball on Earth and it doesn't go very far - gravity yanks it down, and air resistance slows it the whole way. A few seconds later it's just sitting there in the grass.

Let's talk about your inertia. Or rather, *inertias*, because you have a lot of different moving and unmoving things in your life.

So in both instances - the unmoving rock and bag, and the moving baseball - are examples of inertia.

So now we are on the same real page.

134

Some people mistakenly call that momentum; it's *not*. It's *inertia*, and it's a perfectly applicable description of how we move through life - metaphorically.

Your inertia

Let's talk about your inertia. Or rather, *inertias*, because you have a lot of different moving and unmoving things in your life.

Everything in your life has inertia. There are things that have no motion: they just sit there, anchored to your life the way the rock is anchored to the earth.
There are things that are in motion, like the baseball that keeps moving depending on how many external elements start messing with it.

Things in motion in your life

Your job - you get up for work every day at about the same time and do what you need to do to be there. If it's a job then you probably predictably go home at the same time. If it's a career then you predictably do NOT go home at the same time, and so forth. It's in motion.

The same is true for your relationship - it is in motion, you see your significant other at a certain rhythm or rate. You give it a certain amount of time in your life - a certain amount of effort, and you fit it in with the other things.

Things at rest in your life

There are things in your life that are at rest - they don't move, they don't do nothin'. You may say that if they don't move at all they aren't even in your life. But they are. There are things in your life that used to move, but no longer do - things like a workout class you no longer attend because you have kids now. Or a fun hobby you no longer do because you don't have the time, or the energy to do it any more. Or you used to date, but now you figure it's just too much effort and being alone is easier. They all sit there, some are like rocks, and some are closer to feathers. Most are probably rocks if you've already forgotten about them. It will take a lot of time and energy to get that hobby going again, until then it's just sitting in the ground. See how it works in both directions? You can have a rock that will take a lot of effort to start up, or a rock that will take a lot of effort to end - like a relationship you are just comfortable in, or a bad habit you can't seem to break.

Awareness

There are a lot of things in your life in motion, and at rest - in fact more than you are aware of. It's this lack of awareness that keeps them in their current state. In some cases it's convenient, in other cases it's not only *not* convenient but kind of harmful. Creating an awareness - or heightening your awareness - of these things can only help.

Your Homework

Spend a few minutes thinking about what is *at rest* in your life. Think about all the rocks first. What things are just sitting there and there's NO way they are gonna move, except for the metaphorical hurricane or worse. Think about the things you used to do, the things you used to be a part of.

Think about both good and bad.

Then think about all the feathers. Think about those same kind of things, but not the ones that are so rooted. What about the ones that you could start up again, or rather might just start up on their own due to external forces. Good and bad.

This is not an exercise to make you feel guilty or beat yourself up. <u>Don't beat yourself up</u>. You should be as tired of me saying that as you are of me saying "Time, Energy and Resources™!"   The purpose is awareness only.

Formula for managing the rocks and feathers in your life:

- Consider what it would take to get the good rocks moving that you want to move (think working out, or the career you actually wanted)
- Be thankful for the bad rocks that are sitting there and will never move again (think lack of addictions, think lack of anger, think respect for yourself though diet, etc)
- Be aware of why the bad feathers get going again - they got blown around by an external force that messes with you (think over doing drinking and holidays or over eating and being in a hurry)
- Be aware of the good feathers and how potentially flimsy they are

RESTING AND TENSION

Cutting the grass and sump pump hoses

My son came by for the weekend recently and like a good dad I put him to work. He cut the grass for me, and as he was cutting it I moved the sump pump hose out of the way into a position that was temporary - temporary because that's not where I wanted the water to exit. I waited a while for him to cut the area so I could put it back. He kept cutting but not in the same way I would as I would cut the area that the hose was in first so I could put it back. When I started to get amusingly frustrated I said to myself - "That's OK, he doesn't know the resting and tension positions of that hose."

Resting and tension?

Everything has rest and tension. I have not done any research into this but it sounds like a suspiciously ancient Oriental concept - sort of like yin and yang. So I will naively continue. My son couldn't tell that the hose being in that temporary position was a position of "tension" for me. To him it was just a hose we moved. For me, however, it bothered me; it was a tension I could feel. Because if we left it there the water that was ejected would be too close to the house and end up in my basement.   Strange, huh?

Tension

Tension is the feeling that something is not right - that it is out of place or it is in a position that you want to change. It bothers you. It unnerves you; it disturbs you and even drives you crazy. Some of these things are things we just "get used to." Others are things that we just are not at ease with until we truly "put them back" like the innocuous hose. Every day we encounter things in our life that provide tension. In some cases they are the things we are bothered by, in others they are a life adjustment, in others they are just things we need to accomplish and still others are things that we actually have fun changing.

Unnerving and disturbing things are such things as a pay cut, a new boss or policy change that is going to make you quit, a significant other than is constantly bumping heads with you and on the way out, a teenager that is out of control or even a bunch of weight gain. These are all things that you feel you cannot change or are very difficult to change.

Things you may not be at ease with are a messy living room, a pile of laundry that needs to be done, if you live in Wisconsin then it's the four-foot snow drifts that completely prevent any means of escape. All these things can be changed and you know how to change them.

Then there are the little things - the stuff they tell you (inaccurately) not to "sweat." These are things like emptying the dishwasher, taking a shower, writing an email or the aforementioned hose - all tension in your universe.

Finally there are the things you want to change, and are looking forward to changing - things like a work out you're looking forward to, a painting you are working on, sculpting, pottery work, home improvements, a carwash, even coding.

Resting

The things at rest in your life are the things that seem to be where you want them. When you review these they give you a certain kind of contentment. Things that are at rest are not necessarily things that are not moving. This is not an inertia or momentum discussion like we had in the "Rocks and Feathers" chapter. Whether the thing is maintained or is on autopilot is not a function of whether you consider it resting. A high school coach that is watching his team run sprints has a lot of movement in front of him. He has to maintain their activity level, watch for stragglers, for form, etc. They are in no way "resting" nor is he at the moment - but the activity itself, the flow of it in his mind is considered resting.

Whether the thing is maintained or is on autopilot is not a function of whether you consider it resting.

Things at rest in your life could be the health you happily maintain though good eating an exercise. You may consider a clean and very tidy house to be at rest, and conversely you may consider a house with toys strewn about to also be at rest because you are the parent of small kids and this state of being means they are happy and your house is alive with movement and happiness. Your concept of resting may be connected to whether you are someone who favors order or chaos - both could be considered rest or tension depending on your view. Check out "Order or Chaos?" to see which one you are.

A very active office, with many many "balls in the air" could be your state of resting environment. If you paint it could be a canvas in the middle of the studio surrounded by other canvases - paints, brushes, props - so strewn about as to hide the floor completely. Whatever it is, it is in a state that makes you feel like you were meant to do this - you are performing your function. And confusingly, this feeling can come from having something in a state of tension - a completely blank canvas looking very alone in the middle of a clean room, or a blank sheet of paper or blinking cursor on your Mac Pages, beckoning you to start once again.

So don't fault others for not knowing what is causing tension - you may just have to explain it to them with the hope they understand. And understand that others have things that provide tension that may be invisible to you as well.

And don't beat yourself up.

Magic items: Resting and Tension

- Learn which things in your life provide tension and rest

- If you change something does it make you feel better or worse?

- Experiment with small things and they may reveal something they have been hiding

ORDER OR CHAOS

Order or Chaos?

Which are you? Are you all for order, and organization and things being in neat predictable rows? Or do you like things to be all over the place, with no clear order?

Spoiler alert, you are most certainly both.

When we think of order or chaos, we think of the two elements in conflict in the universe. Systems are trying to assemble themselves into neat and orderly patterns. Other bits and pieces are seemingly at random going in all directions pulling that apart.

In your life you will definitely experience and participate in both. However, you will probably tend towards one than the other.

Order

You like order, so you like things to be predictable. You like things to be lined up neatly. The more complex something is the more you want it to be ordered, because this ordered predictability is what helps you deal with the complexity. You like your paperwork to all have nice labels you printed on the label maker, right?

Maybe some color coding in there – all right in the file cabinet? You find yourself being kind of picky about office supplies – you like the nice stuff. And if it all matches somehow even better. You even use this organization need to motivate you to buy things like drawers, storage units, stuff for your office. So what if it's a little more expensive – that's what the organized professionals use.

If you are big on order then your house being in disarray may really get you yelling. All you want from the kids is for them to put their shoes in one place – it doesn't have to look like they exploded and all their clothes went flying, right?

How hard is it to not do that?

Chaos

You find things all lined up to be stifling. Too much of that is just robotic, and what makes you human is your ability to create. In fact, you find this forced order to be the mortal enemy of creativity. After all, writing, painting, photography - they are all produced by people who don't do the same thing and fall in line. The ones that even break the creativity rules (the order *within* the creativity) are the ones that get noticed and set trends.

You're Both, but when?

So, like yin and yang, it is a healthy thing for us to be made of both. And we are. In the examples above you may feel you fit in one, or both. We experience and participate in order and chaos all the time. The question is when, and how it applies to our personalities, and our outlook in life. We may feel that being in a "messy" house means you are human, and that makes us comfortable. Going to a house in which the person keeps it in pristine state all all times bothers you.

On a dating site there is often a question:

Would you date someone who is messy?

Almost all women answer "No" because messy to them (in the specific context of a man) sounds like a slob, a lazy person who may even have bad hygiene.

A lot of men answer "Yes" they would date a messy person because in the context of a woman for them they just imagine it as someone who is human, and isn't too uptight.

Two views of the same thing. In the case of the woman they value the order; in the case of the men it is the chaos that makes it attractive.

You're both. So is everyone. The troubles begin when someone becomes too one-sided. And sometimes the environment perpetuates this.

You may be someone who keeps an impeccably clean and ordered desk at work, but has a house in which things are a bit unordered. For you it is a professional thing – you'd never be caught being chaotic at work because to you chaotic equals unprofessional and that's unacceptable and embarrassing. However, how you keep your home is another thing. It's unrelated to your business and doesn't reflect poorly on you professionally. In fact, a messy house to you means you are a good attentive parent and this messiness speaks to where your attention actually goes.

You're both. So is everyone. The troubles begin when someone becomes too one-sided. And sometimes the environment perpetuates this.

Take the example of the singer/performer who becomes famous.

They have a way of creating – they don't care about order or showering or keeping a clean house. They move around so much – a trailer, hotels, etc. - that all that mundane stuff is offloaded. They feel very strongly that this stuff interferes with their creative process. In fact, fear plays a big part in keeping them chaotic and away from any kind of order. So they go overboard.

Magic items: Order and Chaos

Reflect on what parts of your life are chaotic and what parts are order. Why are they like that? Do they serve you? How does order make you feel? Do you feel control? Responsible? Adult? professional? Do you use order to push back on the world and say "Yeah, I got this."

How does chaos serve you? Do you feel creative? Special? Do you migrate towards others who are chaotic, because that makes them "easy going" and they too like to "stick it to the man?"

You may be surprised at the reasons why you do this. You may have made chaos a security blanket. Order may be used as a shield.

Either way, make sure it serves you.

JOB, CAREER OR CALLING?

We spend a tremendous amount of our lives earning a living - over a third by some estimates. What you do for a living affects your lifestyle, your happiness and your sense of well-being. It is clearly very important.

You chose your job because it was your dream job, wasn't it? OK, perhaps you do it because that's what you went to college for? Ok, well maybe it is something you are just good at?

Maybe you "fell into it" - meaning, at one point you just realized you had been in this job, or at this company for 20 years.

If you'd like to be happy, and content, it's important to know if you have a job, a career or a calling. You may have all three.

Job

A job is the simplest form of work. It's the easiest to obtain and means the least when you lose it. I'm not minimizing the devastation that can occur if someone loses their job after a couple decades, nor am I saying that anyone can get any job. Technically careers and callings are also "jobs."

Let me clarify. If you have a job it means you show up, do your work, and then leave. Once you go home you are done. No one calls, and if you go on vacation you just pick up from where you left off. "Do you want fries with that?" comes to mind when you think of this.

That is not to say a job can't be lucrative, or long term, or fulfilling. Some people are very happy at their jobs and that is all they want - a place to show up, contribute and go home. They lead meaningful, happy lives and their job never gets in the way of that happiness.

That is not to say a job can't be lucrative, or long term, or fulfilling.

Career

Do you spend a lot more than eight hours at work? When you go home do you eat a quick bite and then open your laptop to continue working? Is half of your vacation spent answering emails on your phone? When was the last time you didn't think about work?

If you have a career it usually means that you have immersed yourself in a field and are pursuing that field with considerable commitment. Those in this mode are going to be in this field for the rest of their lives, as far as they know.

Calling

You know if you have a calling. You have this intense desire to do something. You always look and feel happy when you do it. No, eating cookies or drinking wine doesn't count[36]. The first time you heard that word was probably as part of the sentence, "You missed your calling" in which you did something for someone that

---

[36] Well, actually it does. More on that later.

was out of the ordinary for you and they were very impressed. Sometimes it's said as a joke but often it is accurate.

You are told to do what makes you happiest and then find a way to get paid for it.

When we think of a calling we think of people such as singers, performers, pastors, teachers and artists. Each one seems like a vocation for which you would have passion. Unlike careers and jobs not all callings generate income; in fact the monetary compensation is not part of the draw. It is the *act* itself. Pursuing your calling is in many people's opinion the ultimate expression of happiness and freedom. And you are told by many to "find your calling." You are told to do what makes you happiest and then find a way to get paid for it. Seems like reasonable advice, but it is also limiting. Why? Read on and I'll explain.

What do you have?

As I said your happiness can be affected intensely by what you do for a living - not just the chosen field, but your commitment to it. It affects your mood, your concentration, the amount of funds you have, the amount of free time you have and your flexibility. You probably heard the words "time" "energy and "resources" jump out of that sentence, didn't you?

Goals

It is important to have an understanding on where you are with your employment. Each one provides and affects your life differently.

If you work an 80 hour week in the financial field your desire to meet new people, or pursue a new hobby is markedly different than someone who only works 40 hours doing something relatively simple. And the latter person doesn't get calls at 2am.

However, the person with the high-paying career may have the funds necessary to eventually open the mom and pop store they always wanted to have.

No one should pursue goals while completely ignoring what they do for a living, yet many do.

If you tell someone that you really want to learn how to play the violin the first question is never, "Oh, what do you do for a living?" It should be.

Think about that.

That one question is really asking the following:

"How much free time does your job allow you?"

"Does your job provide spendable income that could be used for lessons?"

"Is your job so draining emotionally that even if you had the time you won't have the emotional energy to take lessons and commit to it?"

Obviously there are many factors in making changes to your life[37], but since your work not only takes so much time and energy from you and is the primary source of funding it should be very high on your list.

All the planning in the world is not going to get you to where you want to be if your job is draining the life out of you.

Nor is pursuing an expensive venture if you just don't have (or

---

[37] Which was why I created the balance sheet.

can't get) the funding for it.

Regarding the cookie eating and the wine drinking, two words: Baker and Sommelier.

Alternate routes

By now you probably believe that it is the ultimate thing to have a calling. And if you don't have one then you just aren't as interesting as your friend who does have one. In addition if you know someone who makes a living at their calling then they really hit the jackpot.

It's nonlinear

What you are not considering is that a job, career and path to calling is not linear. For some they may have a job, then a career and then a calling. But for some they are able to do more than one at the same time.

It is perfectly reasonable to work a job so that your calling is funded. Your job is not fulfilling, but it provides a good living for you and doesn't demand much time or energy. You get to go home at the end of the day and you don't work weekends. It's solid. It's an anchor. Because of this anchor you can accumulate the funds to go spend time on your calling - capturing animals, photographically. Perhaps you don't feel you are a world-class photographer, but you are pursuing this calling, it feels amazing and you can afford it. You have a job and a calling *at the same time*.

Will you be discovered in five years and be paid substantially, ludicrously for it? Maybe not, but maybe you will because you had the luxury of allowing your passion to come through - because of your job.

So, before you give up on a passion, or beat yourself up for not having one, consider the above.

Not all artists sculpt something on day one and sell it for the price of a house. Not all writers write The Great American novel and are discovered immediately.

Most overnight successes take ten years.

And success is measured in many ways.

Formula for happiness in employment:

- Use the above to test whether your employment is a job, a career or a calling.
- Give thought to your hobbies and activities, and if any of them seem like a calling
- Think about your happiness in your profession - do you do it because you re good at it, or because you really love it, or both?

THE CANARY DOES NOT MINE COAL

We just talked about jobs, careers and callings.   So before we move on to other things we should talk about the little canary, because he might be you.

You may or may not know this, or you may be just using the metaphor without actually knowing the origin, but have you heard of the canary in the coal mine?

People use the metaphor to describe something or someone who is more sensitive to change than others. They use it to describe an indicator of change, or when things go bad.

It's a real thing. Yes there were canaries in coal mines. This has been done for a century[38].

Because the little canary has tiny sensitive lungs, and breathes in and out many times faster than we do it becomes susceptible to issues in the air before we do. If noxious gases were present in a tunnel, the canary would show signs of distress, go unconscious, even die. This would happen before the miners themselves were in danger, so upon seeing this they would exit the mine. The canary would save them from injuries, even death.

---

[38] This ended as recent as 1986 according to some sources.

But it did not mine coal.

You could make a very solid argument that a group of miners with a canary could focus more on mining coal, be bolder about exploring and generally be much more efficient than one without a canary. Mind you - it's highly unlikely that any mining company would chose not to use one, but I am comparing the presence of the canary to a group without it.

I was - in many respects - their canary.

I tell you all of this because you may either hire or be a canary.

Let me make a quick disclaimer that what I am about to outline is not a job or position that is created as part of a politically correct movement, or a position that doesn't serve a purpose.

They use it to describe an indicator of change, or when things go bad.

My personal experience has been in the 15+ years that I ran a technology consulting service, there were some vital contributions that I made to small and medium-sized businesses. I was behind the scenes in some capacities, and in other times in the forefront. However, what I did for those companies on an ongoing basis helped them to be more efficient, concentrate on their actual business, be more competitive and be aware of technologies that were invisible to competitors.

I was - in many respects - their canary.

If you're the canary

If you are a canary you may focus on your inability to mine coal. You'll look down at your cute little wings and talons - unable to hold a pickaxe. You'll realize that none of the helmets would fit you, and that you contribute no coal to the bins.

Your abilities and most importantly your core talent(s) may make you the canary on your team, or for your clients, or even your family.

Your abilities and most importantly your core talent(s) may make you the canary on your team, or for your clients, or even your family.

So, if you read through *Job, Career or Calling?* and came up a little confused, daunted or even ashamed that you don't have this monumental talent remember these three things:

- Your core talent and contributions - like the canary - may be just as vital even though it is not what the rest of the team does
- You may downplay your core talent because it is not as glorious, public or as common as what everyone else does
- Your core talent(s) may be so unique that finding an application for it may be challenging
- You may need to find your core talent(s)

As I mentioned I felt that I was all over the map until I realized that I was doing the same thing over and over based on my (up until then) unrealized core talent. Yours may be like that - something working hard in the background driving you to do seemingly disparate things.

Don't undervalue your skills, little canary.

Formula for finding your core talents:

- Do you feel different than your team / group / family / tribe?
- Focus on this thing that makes you different - it may be your core talent, or a production of it (see the "My Story" chapter)
- Reflect on how you respond to adversity, to challenges and needs - are they all similar "responses?"
- If the responses all seem unrelated, think about what produced them - what would produce all these seemingly dissimilar responses?

CHARGING A BATTERY, FILLING A MUG, ACCOMPLISHING A GOAL

Charging a battery

We all own devices that run on batteries - iPhones, Androids, laptops, various pads, smart watches, wireless headphones. Charging them sometimes becomes a sport in which we actually change our behavior based on how much time we can get out of a certain item, right? We charge at night, or while we are showering, etc. Ever notice that everything with a battery charges a certain way? It may take three hours to charge something but the way it charges is not linear.

Filling a bucket

It's easy to liken charging to filling up a bucket or mug without spilling. Imagine that your battery is a mug (or your latte, or beer), and the charger's job is to fill it to the very top without spilling.

Spilling some equals ruining the battery (or at least drastically reducing its capacity and effectiveness). If you want to fill this bucket as fast as possible you just dump the water into it and try to stop at the very top. If you pour too much you screwed up the battery (and got the floor all wet). If you stop too soon you underfilled the bucket (and the battery only has 80% of the charge it is supposed to have). So your charger does just what you'd eventually learn to do: **It charges very quickly in the beginning** (it just dumps the water in as fast as possible) **and then slows down near the end**, and just gives it a trickle at the very very end. In fact some charges just sort of stop at 98% and then wait until it falls below 94%. They play it safe.

Accomplishments and goals

Accomplishments and goals are very similar to this battery and bucket. In fact, this charging method is a perfect metaphor for how goals are sometimes accomplished (and not).

This is also why no one erects a statue to a committee.

Remember the last thing you tried to accomplish? No, not doing the dishes - something larger like a project or even a major goal. You probably plunged into it full-force, and got a great start. As the project progressed and you became aware of the many steps and milestones and sub-tasks needed... you slowed down. Maybe it wasn't voluntary - after all if you were working and depending on others you may have had to wait for them.* But indeed you slowed down. As you approached the finish line a few things may have happened:

The goal changed - once you were deep into the goal/ accomplishment you discovered/realized a few things you were ignorant of before starting. So the goal line moved. The battery has more capacity than you thought or the bucket is deeper. *So your trickle at the end is a trickle at the middle.*

You lost interest/became daunted - This can happen when the minutia of the task eats you up. A death by 1,000 cuts is a very real pitfall of accomplishing a goal** You can also lose interest because, *hey, I didn't know it would be like this* and *jeez, this is harder than I thought* and *maybe this isn't for me.* **I don't really want to charge this battery, maybe someone else should do it?**

You get paralysis by analysis - This is also why no one erects a statue to a committee. Though analysis is important if that's all you're doing you're not moving forward. *So your charging is really looking at the battery, wondering about the best charger to use, or maybe considering filling the bucket with something other than water.*

You want to do it right - you look back at your progress and you really become one with the moment, being aware of the shift of time. *This battery is going to be charged perfectly to 100%, and that bucket is gonna get filled to the very top. Also, good beer, and fine latte.*

You start to savor the victory - a wonderful but dangerous thing to do, akin to counting those chickens before they are hatched. *You may become so busy celebrating the 85% progress of the bucket fill and battery charge that it never goes higher.*

The next time you order a latte or a beer, watch how it is poured quickly in the beginning and then slowly at the end.

Be mindful

So, be mindful that the process of charging a battery, filling a bucket and accomplishing a major goal has a certain method for a reason. The next time you order a latte or a beer, watch how it is poured quickly in the beginning and then slowly at the end. It can be a great reminder of how you can and should accomplish your goals. And if you associate the pleasure of having a latte or a beer with accomplishing a goal, that's even better. See "F.L.A.T." on what I mean by that. I know you already read it though.

I want your battery to be charged to 100% and your bucket to be filled to the very top - because there's going to be another battery and another bucket soon, and they'll be even larger. Or in your case, maybe a beer.

* *My experience with web development has taught me that the major delays and slowdowns of producing a newly developed site is mostly caused by waiting for the client to decide on an option, or deliver needed media.*

** *Writing a book is not just creating a manuscript - there are many tiny things that need to happen properly that have little or nothing to do with the creative process. But you still have to do 'em.*

Formula for navigating a long-term goal:

- Be mindful of where you are in the process
- When you get near the end expect a change in how you go about finishing
- Be mindful of the change ion speed
- Be mindful that the goal you originally shot for may not be the actual goal - that's OK

DREAD AND DOUBT

I read a lot of articles on productivity, personal development and all that jazz. More accurately, I naively see a great title, start to read the article, and then find it's the same thing over and over. I've learned that the more the title promises, the more the article disappoints. I've learned that the title is like a label on a bottle, and that the article is the actual formula. There are a lot of labels promising eternal youth, a cure for what ails you and super strength. There are article titles telling you that if you just do these two things something remarkable happens. They tell you that they have something astounding to tell you, and that in just few paragraphs you'll have this tidbit of wisdom that will Change Your Life Forever.

The raising and the dashing

Over and over again, my hopes are raised by just a few words and then four minutes later dashed on the craggy rocks below – shattered and disbursed by the crashing waves that laugh as they smash into whatever little fragments of hopes are left, absorbing them into the salty cold waters below.

Such is the life of someone searching for answers, unabashedly open to the wisdom of others.

So, you can imagine how I approach doing the same thing: making a promise in a title and then delivering something tangible in the body. My labels may not be as exciting with New and Improved and You've Never Seen This Before but the formula is solid.

Two things make a huge difference

When I say these two things will make a huge difference, I mean it. When I say I've identified a cork that you can pull out to allow stuff to happen I mean it. And I'm not asking for you to Try This For Only 200 Days. **No, try it for a *day*. Try it in the morning, see what happens *an hour later*.** Yeah, I made that bold because you're lazy and were just skimming. Ha. Gotcha.

Dread

Motivational people talk about a lot of things. I'm just going to talk about two things I've identified that make a big difference – this time we will deal with dread.

Dread is the feeling that you don't want to do something. When you think about it you say "ugh" and have this flight or fight reaction. More accurately it's a leave-your-house, do-something-else, procrastinate reaction. Maybe tomorrow, oh look it's Friday how about Monday?

We have *all* done this, a number of times.

Doubt is when you are unsure of your actions. It is not so much that you are unsure of the outcome; you are actually just unsure that you are doing the right thing. Since you can't seem to figure out what the right thing is (due to your feelings of inadequacy, or lack of information, or feeling that the person you are dealing with is just so nuts) you shake your head and essentially freeze. It's paralysis by analysis.

People who write motivational books focus on doubt. They tell

172

you to execute, they tell you that it is all in the follow through, they tell you that this basketball player made x number of shots but missed x * 1,000 shots too. They tell you that you miss 100% of the shots you don't take. That's exhausting just reading that.

But you can't just *tell* someone to stop doubting, because you're ignoring the *reason* for the doubt, silly. And if you don't ignore the *reason* you might end up imparting tangible useful items to your readers/listeners.

Imagine that.

Here's what to do about dread

So here's what to do. You don't need to do it for a year, or a month, or a week. You can actually try it one morning. This will only work on a day that you are experiencing dread and or doubt, though. If you aren't then there's nothing to do. So, on a day that you are dreading something, doubting what to do in a situation or both do the following.

Take a breath and allow yourself to feel the dread, just let it wash over you so that you can fully agree that you are dreading a thing. Yes *really*. You have to feel it for this to work. Focus on what the thing is. Is it talking with a client, or an employee, your boss, spouse, boyfriend or teenager? Now that you know what you are dreading, ask yourself why. That should be obvious – "Because they will yell at me!" "Because they are so crazy and this will just explode and get worse," "Because they always react negatively." "Because…"

Now take the next step. Play it out in your mind. When you do this thing, do you feel that it is the proper thing to do? In other words, are you doing what *you feel is right in the situation*?
Yes? I'm pausing here because it's important. You have to play it out and believe that what you are doing is the right thing. Take your time and feel it.

Once you agree that what you are doing is correct, and not fueled or tainted by things like spite, anger, disrespect or other things that are not who you really are – you can then play out their reaction.

You've now removed any guilt, bad feelings and anything else that divided you about this interaction.

One of two things will now happen. Because the person controlling the play in your head (you) is on board with what you are doing, you will see the interaction in your head as being less emotional and more normal. You may even see the other person reaction a bit more plausibly and realistically.

"Huh, that's not a big deal, that is the right thing and oh well if they don't like it, it really is reasonable," your brain says.

Now, go back to the feeling of dread. Is it still there? Or did it dissolve? If I'm right, then it dissolved[39].

What is doubt?

Doubt is supposed to be a "feeling of uncertainty or lack of conviction." Sounds simple enough, right? If you doubt something then you're uncertain, or not really into it. Well, doubt wouldn't be such a big deal if that's all it was – it's a lot more than that. And more importantly, it's what it does to you, your schedule and your day.

Here's what to do about doubt

So here's what *not* to do. Don't just shove yourself into it. Don't just "try" and think "Oh well better just jump in with both feet" and other motivational cliches. No, instead it's another mental/emotional exercise.

---

[39] Results with myself and others show that the vast majority who do this have most of not all dissolve.

Again set the stage and play it through on your stage. You do this thing and... what happens? Chances are the world doesn't end. There are usually two versions of what happens next:

You run into the wall of *I Don't Know What's Going To Happen, that's the problem!* Ahh. You are afraid of the outcome to the point that you just pull the curtains. The actors just stand there. There's no more to the script. Well that's not helpful, is it? Nope. So do this instead: Since it's just a stage in your head open those curtains and when they say "line" tell them. And watch. Watch what happens because your answer of "I have no idea" is like poop to me. You DO know. You have enough experience with humans, young and old, crazy and sane, to have a clue and play it out. So play it out. Now play it out again and change it a little. Now change it again. Did this one seem absurd? Did you feel that it's just dumb to think that this would be the outcome? Good, then pull back and do it again.

You're playing with the permutations and possibilities. In other words, you're both getting in touch with the actual reality, and your understanding of it. It's both of those things being off that causes the doubt in the first place.

Now do it a final time. Oh, you're bored? Why? Because its... *obvious* that this is how it will work? Then you have done well. Stop judging the article and do it.

"But I'm really bad at [That Thing] and that's why I have the doubt, you dummy," you think and/or say.
Ok, if you're sure about that then nothing will change when you run through the simulation above right? I'll wait.

If it did change, then you see how doubt masquerades as knowledge, or lack thereof.

If it didn't change, then it revealed what you're not certain about, or why you're uncertain, and that helps you do solve that and come back.

In conclusion

If you're the average person, and were experiencing doubt and/or dread, and have truly gone through this simple simulation then you probably no longer feel it.

It's pretty cool, isn't it?

Formula to remove doubt:

On a day that you are feeling doubt, take a few minutes to play the scenario in your head like a stage you control. Play through the situation snd question how absurd the outcome is. Play it over a few times until the outcome seems more reasonable.

You will:

- Reveal an absurdity you created
- Feel more in line with your core beliefs (since you are not a jerk, and not acting out, then you will have more confidence in the correctness of your actions)
- Create a possibility more in line with reality

Formula to remove dread:

On a day that you are experiencing doubt, create a stage in your mind similar to the above. Play out the outcome. Again, play it out a few times until the outcome reveals the most likely end. Give the actors their lines instead of just giving up. it is the giving up that creates the doubt.

IN THE ZONE

In The Zone

Have you ever been "in the zone?" Have you ever heard someone say "I'm in the zone, don't bother me?" If you have then you know what I am talking about. If you've never really been in the zone then let me explain, because this is a really amazing thing, and you need to not only know about it, but you need to experience this as often as you can.

Defining it

I did a lot of searching to see what others thought the definition was. The one I found that was closest to my perception is the definition by the Collins English Dictionary – a dictionary I hadn't heard of until now.

In the zone
Informal
In a state that produces achievement with
such an extraordinary, often unlikely,
degree of success that
it seems to defy purely rational
explanation.

It is interesting that it mentions an "often unlikely" degree of success, isn't it? You are doing something that seems to produce an achievement, with a very satisfying and unusual degree of success that you can't seem to explain. I think that's a big part of it. You go to do something - to create something - and when done you look at what you've done and marvel at the outcome – *dang that turned out really really well*.

That's a part of it, but let's take an even larger view and encompass the entire concept - in my humble opinion of course.

Not only do you feel like you're good at this, but you just feel *right* doing it.

Being in the zone just feels right. It feels like you are doing something you are good at – something you are exceptional at. That feeling of perceiving that you are very good at it is a feeling of *self-validation*. And we all know just how powerful validation is – it's the feel-all be-all emotion. But the zone is more than that.

The second facet - it feels right

If you were good at something but didn't like it then you would only have a two-dimensional feeling of validation. The other facet adds another dimension. Not only do you feel like you're good at this, but you just feel *right* doing it. When you do this you feel like *this is your thing*. This is your domain. Hold my beer. It's the third act and you are up. That's a really important part – that feeling that you are doing your thing. This acts as a self-contained fuel for the validation. You do the thing and enjoy it, then take a step back and say "Dang Karen, you really are good at this!" But wait, there's more.

The third facet - validation

There's a third facet of The Zone. This facet is not required but it just makes the zone that much easier to attain for some, and it involves the V word again. Again, you do this thing, then you look upon it and pronounce it amazing, this validating yourself and fueling your passion for it. But now you show it to others and *they* go crazy over it - not only confirming your assessment of it, but increasing the assessment to another level. You think it's great – humbly and almost secretly – and they all think it is awesome! Now you have external validation that adds to your fuel.

What is your zone?

There's no limit as to what your zone is. It can be writing, acting, creating music, your specific form of art, or even playing Santa. it can be something everyone else thinks is mundane - crunching numbers on a spreadsheet, cleaning your bathroom, preparing lunches for your kids for school, driving , writing proposals, coding or Christmas shopping.

The act doesn't matter; the feeling does.

Discovering your gages

If you follow me and are aware of *The Status Game* then you're aware of how you're guided by these gages on your dashboards. If you haven't been in The Zone then that's a crime. **You need to find your zone**.

Formula for being in The Zone:

Be mindful of how you feel when you are participating in something that get's you excited. Think about your personal, subjective view at how good you are at a task. Have you shown this task to others, thus testing the third facet?

If you have learned that this task or activity is what puts you in the zone, have you pursued it further? Have you attempted to change it from a casual occurrence to a hobby or even a career? Perhaps it is your calling.

NEW YEAR'S RESOLUTIONS

Happy New Year

New years resolutions are so common that they deserve their own area of this book. In fact, for most people a new year's resolution is the only contact they have with even thinking about a goal, or making a change in their lives.

Once a year they make their resolutions, state them proudly, and go about their lives. Most never think of them again.

New years resolutions are a way to make yourself feel better... in December.

According to Wikipedia, about half of the US makes New Year's Resolutions each year. Another study of 3,000 people sampled showed that 88% of those who set new years resolutions *fail*. 88%. That's about nine people out of ten. That's a lot of failure.

In fact, for most people a new year's resolution is the only contact they have with even thinking about a goal, or making a change in their lives.

Why all the fail?

The most common reason for participants failing their New Year's Resolutions was setting themselves unrealistic goals (35%), while 33% didn't keep track of their progress and a further 23% forgot about it. About one in 10 respondents claimed they made too many resolutions. Regardless of the breakdown, the overarching reason for failure is essentially the same – setting a goal. But how can you have success if you don't set a goal? Isn't balance coaching all about setting goals and achieving them? And for that matter, isn't all coaching just setting goals?

All very valid questions

A goal is an end point; a thing you can check off. It's great for little things; for small pieces of a larger whole. It's great as a marker, a milestone. It's great in things that keep score, like sports, or in some cases weight loss.

It's not great in cases where you are making a life long change, or measuring less tangible things, or when considering health as a whole.

A resolution is like a checkmark next to a word. There's a difference between *I'm going to do X* and saying you are going to *accomplish a thing*. If you want to accomplish a thing, you have to step back and realize there is a system involved.

So, in accomplishing this thing you not only have to develop some sort of system to do it, you have to make the room in your Time, Energy and Resources.

If you're lucky, after a little introspection you decide it would be a good thing to give up something, or do something more, or commit time to a thing, or somehow produce a thing out of thin air.

You resolve to do it…

In the beginning it works because every day it's on your mind. Every day you say "Oh yeah, no more coffee" or "Eat better" or "Eat more salad" or you join a gym, but you don't know when you'll go. You just try to go as often as you can. For a few days you sort of feel good, but the reality of it sinks in.

…and then you don't.

If you don't make this room all the planning and good intentions will not make it happen. And, as I've said, if you don't make the room it will be forcibly ejected from your Time, Energy and Resources. It will be rejected by your *schedule* "I just didn't have the time - that was crazy to try to make it to practice every Wednesday." It will be rejected by your *energy* - "I'm just not cut out for that sort of thing, I'm too old, or it's just not right for me." It will be ejected from your *resources* - "That's too expensive, I guess I'm not rich enough to be fit."

Does that sound painfully familiar?

If that makes sense then why would you believe that you can just set a goal and do one thing the entire time?

Steering from afar

Imagine that you have a pretty simple car - no cool GPS or anything. There is a city pretty far away - perhaps over 100 miles away. Even though it is that far away you can still see it, barely. You can see the buildings there - all clumped together and shrouded mostly in mist.

There are a few roads but you can also drive off road because things are pretty flat.

You want to go to the city so you just point your car at it, and go.

The car doesn't have autopilot but you can just lock the steering wheel in "straight ahead." What do you think happens eventually?

Eventually you see that you are not pointed exactly at the city. You're not even halfway there and you can tell you are going to miss the city by miles, to the left. Under normal circumstances you would just make a course correction, right? Just adjust the wheel slightly to the right, keep going, maybe tilt slightly to the left. Repeat until you reach the city. You know: steering.

If that makes sense then why would you believe that you can just set a goal and do one thing the entire time?

Your path to the goal will need some course corrections along the way. A little to the left, a little to the right. When you adjust the steering wheel on the car you don't beat yourself up and think "What was I thinking?" No, you just adjust. Why? Because you know how inaccurate it is to steer from afar.

The farther away from the city, the more likely you are going to miss it if you don't make adjustments.

No, you just adjust. Why? Because you know how inaccurate it is to steer from afar.

So if the city is your goal, the car is you and the distance is your journey you will need to do the same thing.

When you set a goal that's not just a checkbox; you have to realize that you are pointing your car at it from pretty far away. If it's January 1st and your goal is to lose 50 pounds, there's going to be a lot of steering involved. It's highly unlikely that you lose those pounds by going about your life normally, and just giving up one item.   It's more likely that you lose 10 pounds quickly but then find it's harder to lose the rest. Or, as you are losing weight you start to become less interested in the final number, but more interested in the pleasing shape your body is taking. Or you really like the competitive cardio that you are doing, and you've made new friends - friends that are a good influence in your life because they have the healthy attitude you want.

So, not only to you make lots of corrections, you decide that you don't want to go to the 50 pounds weight loss city but instead the one with new friends, healthier body and fun competitive cardio.

That's something most people don't consider when making a resolution - that they are planning something so absolute from so far away, and that they may learn things on the way that will change their actual goal.

It's a wonderful thing, because the new goal is almost always better than the knee-jerk, I'm-so-fed-up resolution that is made in frustration.

...they are planning something so absolute from so far away, and that they may learn things on the way that will change their actual goal.

The new goal is a better fit for your life, comes with an added bonus and is part of a learning process.

I'm not saying that there's anything wrong with setting a definitive goal and reaching it - people do that all the time.

Just be mindful that setting a goal that's really an outcome of "I will be 50 pounds lighter" involves a lot more changes than you think, and it may not even be what's best for you. Imagine that.

I always say "Resolutions are bad" because it generates a strong emotional reaction and gets people thinking.

It's a wonderful thing, because the new goal is almost always better than the knee-jerk, I'm-so-fed-up resolution that is made in frustration.

Formula for making proper New years Resolutions:

- Setting a long-term goal is very much like pointing your car at a far away city; you'll eventually have to make course corrections
- When you make course corrections know that they are part of the process - they are a good thing, not a bad thing
- If you don't make the room in your Time, Energy and Resources your goal is not going to happen - except in the most extreme of life-changing events that will force your hand
- Systems, not goals. If you have a system built around your success it greatly increases your chance of success
- There are some goals that are a simple check box, but you probably wouldn't make them as a new years resolution
- Any movement in a positive direction is a good thing

FAILURE

Hi. Welcome to the last chapter. Contrary to the title I am ending this book on a very positive note.

We have all had failures in our lives, and in fact will continue to do so.

When I was married I wasn't really allowed in the kitchen to help. No, I'm not kidding. Even though I think I would have made an excellent sous chef, I was told that "It's the only thing I'm better at than you and you're just going to get really good at it."

So, when I got divorced and had to cook for my kids, I was very concerned with not killing them through undercooked meats and stuff like that.

Slowly I got better, and then started experimenting with recipes.

Then I started baking. Though I think I was getting pretty darn good at cooking, my baking was very rudimentary. And that's when I learned two big lessons.

Chemistry vs. Alchemy

You see, when you cook and make mistakes you can recover from these mistakes. There are all sorts of tricks you can do if you've overcooked something, or the dish is too spicy, or something is too thick, or not thick enough. You can make changes after the fact.

Cooking is like Alchemy[40].

When you are baking, things are more absolute. Not only do things have to be added in the right proportions, but in the right order. And if you mess things up it's really hard to recover. Most often you are screwed.

Baking is like Chemistry.

When I would bake I would meticulously, fearfully, follow the directions. When I would cook and follow the recipe and it would turn out I would think "great!" But I didn't learn anything. If I cooked and screwed up, I would learn something - especially if it wasn't in the recipe. Replacing one veggie for another, adding a topping to a home made pizza at the last minute instead of with everything, etc.

I learned a lot from my failures. I'm sure you have too.

I learned a lot from my failures. I'm sure you have too. The problem is that we tend to just bury those memories, set rules to avoid pain and move on. But there are things we have failed at that not only taught us lessons, but showed us just how much effort we have put into something.

I interviewed a lovely young woman on my podcast. She told me about a poster she had on her wall. It wasn't a list of successes, but

---

[40] I love that word.

a list of failures. I thought the concept was so fascinating I thought a lot about what failures really were, and the importance of tracking them.

That record shows where your efforts have gone, what the outcomes have been, your stamina and your tenacity.

As I (and many others) have said, an overnight success takes about ten years. In those ten years there are a lot of failures. That record shows where your efforts have gone, what the outcomes have been, your stamina and your tenacity.

A list of your failures can actually be as motivating if not more motivating than your successes.
So, wouldn't it be a great record to go back ten years (or more) and list your failures?

Creating your list of failures

Think about the things you have tried in the past. If you're the kind of person who picks up (and makes it through 200+ pages of) a self-help book then you are most certainly someone who has probably tried many things in life. Some of these things have been minor; some of them have been major. Some have probably been sort of crazy[41].

Once you succeeded you forgot about the failures.

The point is that you put the effort into it, and you may have failed at something multiple times until you understood the right way to

---

[41] I stood in line for three hours, in the middle of summer, in downtown Milwaukee in a suit for the chance to be an extra in Transformers III. And no, I wasn't good enough to be an extra.

do it and succeeded.

Once you succeeded you forgot about the failures.

Or all those failures helped you to understand that you needed to make a course correction[42].

Another interesting thing about failures is that we tend to remember the fail as if it was just a moment - one single moment of pain. We forget all the learning along the way.

Please use the worksheet to proudly record your failures. It is a great reminder and testament to your stamina, your commitment to change, and your unique journey. Trust me - you'll feel pretty good when you look back on it. And, you can look at it any time you are feeling daunted. You can say, "Man, I did all that and didn't give up."

And...

"If I could try that then I can do *this*."

---

[42] Remember the "Steering from afar" chapter?

Formula for embracing failures to energize success:

- List your failures in the past, even if they seem small, or clearly were "off course"
- Review the failures to see a pattern
- Review the failures to appreciate the effort you have put into succeeding - this will allow you to see the effort and not just the result
- You will probably see at least one failure that lead directly to success

WORKSHEETS

These worksheets are included to help you interact with the chapters of this book. Reading about concepts is the start. When you start interacting and recording things in your own words, about your own life, you then take the next step towards getting what you want.

The worksheets are listed with the name of the chapter they reference and a short paragraph as a refresher on the worksheet intentions.

Ultimately reading the preceding chapters and then immediately filling out the worksheets should bring a lot of things to light for you. In some cases they are items you've never given any thought to.

Failure

Think about the failures you've had. Some have been big, some small. Some you repeated - that's important because it means you wanted it, it was in-line with what you wanted, or you were barking up the wrong tree.

<u>Instructions</u>:

- List as many as you care to list
- Be specific on the item line (e.g "applied to be an extra for Transformers III, stood in line and had the photo taken but thats it.")
- Look for patterns
- You should list a failure even if you ended up having success the next time to attempted it, because that failure shows you that this wasn't the end of the road, and that we have failures before we have successes sometimes - "third times the charm"

My Failures

1. _____

_____

2. _____

_____

3. _____

_____

4. _____

_____

5. _____

_____

6. _____

_____

7. _____

_____

8. _____

_____

9. _____

_____

10._____

_____

Comfort Zones

We all have comfort zones. One person's comfort zone is another person's hell. Seriously. You may be in the 2% of the population that feels comfortable speaking in public (like me) or you might be normal like everyone else and would rather have a tax audit and root canal at the same time.

What is important for this worksheet is that you become aware of a comfort zone. If you know that a certain activity, location or way of being is a comfort zone, then you know that it may be exerting a lot of control over you - or preventing you from moving out of it.

Understand that being in an abusive relationship - as horrible and absurd as that sounds - is a comfort zone for some people.

Instructions:

List three comfort zones if possible.

My Comfort Zone(s)

Location / Behavior / Thing

_____

Why is it comfortable?

_____

Location / Behavior / Thing

_____

Why is it comfortable?

_____

Location / Behavior / Thing

_____

Why is it comfortable?

_____

Charging a battery

You have probably found that the when you get close to completing a goal things seem to change - the goal - though closer - is harder to get to. Brute force makes way for finesse.

Just like the barista, or the bartender, or the battery charger you risk not completing the task the way you wanted if you don't make these changes at the end.

Have you ever set a goal but never completed it? Everyone has.

If you get close to a goal but fail to complete it you may write it off as unattainable, or even worse - you'll believe you simply can't do it. The truth is that as you get closer you have to course-correct, apply more concentration, or even have a different finishing approach.

You can do it, you just didn't know this.

Instructions:

List at least one goal you attempted but never reached. How close did you get to it? Write down what you think caused you to stop. It may be an aha moment.

Goals not reached

Goal

_____

How close did you get?

_____

What was the cause?

_____

Goal

_____

How close did you get?

_____

What was the cause?

_____

Order or Chaos?

We are all a bit of order and chaos. Some of us are mostly one of those - and that can be a problem. It seems to be a bit healthier to be a mix of both than to be exclusively one.

Some careers are served rather well by a devotion to one, e.g. - order certainly helps being in the finance sector.

It is important to be aware of your order and chaos because one of them may be getting in the way of your happiness. One of them may be pulling you to the dark side - where your next hobby, career, calling or happiness resides.

Instructions:

List a few activities in your life and label whether they are order or chaos. Then decide whether you are happy with this order (does it ground or stifle you) or chaos (does it make you feel like you're crazy or does it fuel you).

The order and chaos in my life

THING	ORDER / CHAOS?	GOOD /BAD?

Multitasking

Multitasking is not what people think it is. You may be expending more energy than you think you're saving, and becoming more stressed in the process. You may also have found some brilliant ways to cut down on Time, Energy and even Resources.

Instructions:

List at least one pair of items you think you are awesome at doing at the same time. List at least one pair of things you do at the same time that you are terrible at, or at least suffer through. Then circle whether you love it or hate it.

My multitasks

Thing One

_____

Thing Two

_____

Love it!   Hate it!

Thing One

_____

Thing Two

_____

Love it!   Hate it!

Thing One

_____

Thing Two

_____

Love it!   Hate it!

Inertia - Rocks and Feathers

Things in your life take energy to start and stop. Some of them are firmly rooted and we call them "rocks." Some are easy to change and we call them "feathers." Some are good and some are bad.

For most people their diet and exercise level are rocks and hard to change.

Some hobbies are easy to start; some habits are hard to break. It will help you to move forward if you know which is a rock and which is a feather. Obviously you will know which is good and which is bad - at least in your opinion.

Rocks and Feathers can be *anything*.

Instructions:

List a few rocks and feathers in your life and whether they are things you consider to be good or bad.

My Rocks and Feathers

THING	ROCK/ FEATHER?	GOOD/ BAD?

The Canary does not mine coal

You may be part of a team and be the odd man[43] out, or you may have a team member who is. And by "team" we mean any group, which includes families too.

The canaries sometimes forget just how important they are. We don't want that - especially if that's you, little bird. If it's not it will give you a greater appreciation for the bird you know.

Instructions:

List group, canary name, function and why it is so important to the group.

You can list multiple canaries, or even list yourself multiple times if you are the canary for more than one group.

---

[43] Or woman, etc.

The Canaries I know (me?)

Canary / Group

_____ / _____

What is the canary's strength?

_____

Why is this important to the group?

_____

Canary / Group

_____ / _____

What is the canary's strength?

_____

Why is this important to the group?

_____

The Five Facets

Life is made of three things, and we spend them on five.

This is a scaled down, static version of the Alchemy for Life™ site balance sheet used for coaching. It is not included in this book because scaling the sheet down to fit makes it unusable. You can however find it on-line and print

Instructions:

List your activities in each column. You may find that you have none for one of the columns, or that one column contains most of the stuff you do.

Additional worksheets can be found at:

http:www.alchemyfor.life/balancecoaching/worksheets/

The balance sheet is not included in this book because scaling the sheet down to fit makes it unusable. You can however find it online and print it. It is ideally to be used as an interactive sheet[44].

The password[45] for the password-protected worksheets is:

coachme

---

[44] The interactive balance sheet is available as part of a coaching engagement.

[45] Worksheet availability may be limited by time - in other words this worksheet and password may not be valid years after this book is published.

THE AFL PODCAST

Striving to get a handle on life, understanding, gaining wisdom and picking yourself up from a fall is an ongoing thing. As I've said mistakes = pain and pain = experience and experience = wisdom. Every Sunday I try to impart some of those pains turned experience upon the people who are kind enough to listen.

…or if you have an iPhone simply ask Siri, "Hey Siri, play the Alchemy for Life Podcast."

I also find really interesting people and interview them about how they spend their time, energy and resources. In fact, I'm rather obsessed about that. After all, I really wonder how someone gets to a certain point in their life, or how someone finds the energy to accomplish something, or how they dealt with change. Everyone has they own story, and if they have exceedingly unusual circumstances then it makes it even more interesting.

I've interviewed a gentleman who has had a double lung and heart transplant, and then went on to run marathons (three at last count I believe). A woman who is literally a rocket scientist who then went on to write sci-fi - lots of it.   She also watched a shuttle disaster on live TV and realized her friend was on it.   They all have so many stories, and their own way of handling things in their lives.   Mark found the energy to run marathons, Susan started a whole different career being an author.

How did they do it? They clearly had a handle on Time, Energy and Resources.

Listen in for the ten minute podcasts that are similar to the chapters in this book. The interviews are between a half hour and an hour.

Check it out on iTunes, TuneIn, Google Play Music, Spotify, etc.

Just search for "Alchemy for Life podcast" or if you have an iPhone simply ask Siri, "Hey Siri, play the Alchemy for Life Podcast."

Mark Bradford

ABOUT THE AUTHOR

Mark Bradford produces and hosts a weekly podcast about Time, Energy and Resources that also features interviews with amazing people. Listen to *The Alchemy for Life* podcast for more insight, on iTunes and most other podcast providers. Subscribe and you won't miss them.

www.alchemyfor.life

Mark produces *The Status Game* series of books and card game that helps demonstrate, educate and enlighten people about an invisible but very real aspect on how we connect, and what we like.

His answers have over one million answer views on Quora - a question and answer community.

Follow Mark on Instagram for announcements and things related to his content - books, podcasts, etc.

@authormarkbradford

It's a fun feed with daily posts. Have a question?   Ask it on the podcast.

To hire Mark to speak at your event, or engage him as a coach contact him at:

media@alchemyfor.life

Books by Mark Bradford

The Status Game
Navigating the perilous waters of dating and online dating. With a sense of humor.

The Status Game II
How status is the key to all relationships - business and personal.

OneSelf
Faith of a simpler, more direct kind. Or just nonsense.

Alchemy for Life
Everything you need to know about Life Coaching in one book. And 16 formulas for success.

Coming soon:

Three Voices
The languages we use to communicate with others, and ourselves.

Discover Your Gages
The workbook companion to The Status Game II.

Mark Bradford

If you found this book helpful I would appreciate it if you took a minute to review it.

Mark Bradford